One out of [...] workers [...] Find out how to make your job safer.

Cumulative trauma disorders (CTD) of the hands and arms account for almost two-thirds of all job-related illness. They are painful, frustrating, and sometimes disabling.

Most CTD sufferers don't realize that they have been injured until the damage is done. Many doctors aren't trained to recognize the different CTDs, and misdiagnosis is common. The wrong treatment can do more harm than good.

If you work at a computer, as a carpenter, in a butcher shop, on an assembly line . . . *if you work at all,* you have a one in two chance of developing a CTD. This book tells you how to overcome the odds.

*   *   *

"Mark Pinsky has written a book that everyone exposed to Repetitive Strain Injury in the workplace should have by bedside and workside. Those who deal with the problem on an everyday basis may demur with an opinion here or an emphasis there, but *The Carpal Tunnel Syndrome Book* is an invaluable reference for patients and practitioners alike."
—**David J. Eisen, Research & Information Director, The Newspaper Guild (AFL-CIO, CLC)**

"A book for the patient . . . a must for the waiting rooms of all physicians who treat occupational injuries."
—**David M. Pagnanelli, M.D., Chief, Division of Neurosurgery, Abington Memorial Hospital, Abington, PA**

MARK A. PINSKY is the author of *The VDT Book: A Computer User's Guide to Health & Safety* and *Every Citizen's Enviornmental Handbook*. For ten years, he was an editor of *VDT News: The VDT Health and Safety Report*. He has written scores of articles for national publications on CTS, CTDs, ergonomics, and related issues. He has suffered from CTS and from tendinitis, both associated with his computer work.

THE
CARPAL TUNNEL
SYNDROME

BOOK

Preventing and Treating CTS,
Tendinitis and Related Cumulative
Trauma Disorders

Mark A. Pinsky

WARNER BOOKS

A Time Warner Company

The information presented in this book is intended to help you better understand and cope with cumulative trauma disorders of the upper extremities. This book has been reviewed by qualified physicians. It can be a valuable addition to your doctor's advice, and it should be used under his or her care and direction. The author and publisher disclaim all responsibility for any adverse effects resulting from the information contained herein.

This book is not intended as a substitute for medical advice. The reader should regularly consult a physician or health care professional in matters relating to health and particularly in respect to any symptoms that may require diagnosis or medical attention.

WARNER BOOKS EDITION

Copyright © 1993 by Mark A. Pinsky
All rights reserved.

Cover design by Diane Luger
Photographs by Stephen Perloff

Warner Books, Inc.
1271 Avenue of the Americas
New York, NY 10020

 A Time Warner Company

Printed in the United States of America

First Printing: November, 1993

10 9 8 7 6 5 4 3 2 1

TABLE OF CONTENTS

ACKNOWLEDGMENTS

Thanks to Ellen Brown, Marvin Dainoff, Joann Davis, Dr. Larry Fine, Dr. Rutherford Hayes, Colleen Kapklein, Joan Lichterman, Naomi Mindlin, Jennifer Paget, Stephen Perloff, Dr. Linda Pinsky, Al Pinsky, Vern Putz-Anderson, Caroline Rose, and Jerry Sontag.

FOREWORD

This book is not for specialists. It is not for hand surgeons or occupational health specialists who can, and do, draw on volumes of scientific research to understand work-related cumulative trauma disorders (CTDs) of the arms and hands.

This book is for people who need to understand why carpal tunnel syndrome and related disorders occur and what they can do about them. Primarily, it is for the millions of workers who may be at risk of developing CTDs, and for people who already have developed them. It is also for supervisors, managers, and employers, who need to understand what is happening to their employees.

For doctors, it is the sort of book that should be displayed in the waiting room. It encourages patients to prepare thoughtfully for their examinations, and it dispels common misperceptions that patients often bring into the examining room.

With the rising number of cases and the growing recognition that many aspects of modern work are contributing to the development of CTDs, this book fills a critical need for accurate, reliable, sensible, and straightforward information.

Rutherford Hayes, MD
Seattle, WA
February 1993

INTRODUCTION

This book is not just about carpal tunnel syndrome, despite its title. It is a handbook on cumulative trauma disorders (CTDs) that affect the shoulders, arms, elbows, wrists, and hands.

Carpal tunnel syndrome is commonly but incorrectly used as a catchall description for what are technically known as upper extremity CTDs. Because my goal is to inform the underinformed, I chose a title for this book that is imprecise but familiar rather than one that is precise but obscure. Calling this book "The Upper Extremity Cumulative Trauma Disorder Book" would have been an effective way of discouraging potential readers. Those people who already understand the differences among carpal tunnel syndrome, lateral epicondylitis ("tennis elbow"), and stenosing tenosynovitis crepitans ("trigger finger") may object, but then, they don't really need a book like this one.

Awareness is power when your goal is preventing illness on the job. I have written this book with the expectation that readers will use it to improve their health and their working conditions. For different people this will mean different things: The data entry clerk might read how she can adapt her computer work station to reduce the risk of carpal tunnel syndrome. The punch press operator might understand why his arms feel tired so much of the time. The shop foreman might get a fix on what his workers are saying when he hears them talking about ulnar deviations and Raynaud's syndrome. And anyone concerned about the costs of workers' compensation and disability insurance, lost production capacity due to ill workers, and the overall health of our work force will see why the current CTD epidemic is a serious work-related health problem. It is increasingly common to hear job safety specialists describe it as the workplace epidemic of the 1990s.

Most specialists in this field agree that half or more of all American workers—about 65 million people—are at risk for developing one or more CTDs, though a much smaller number will actually develop them. There is every reason to believe that it is significantly less expensive to try to prevent CTDs and to diagnose and treat them aggressively than it is to let CTD cases advance out of control. This book takes the approach that awareness about how to prevent and treat CTDs is what you need most right now. Educate yourself and put your knowledge to work.

Do not expect to eliminate all CTDs simply because you have read this book, or even because you have read all of the supplemental materials listed in the references section at the back of the book. If your job is high-risk—that is, if it involves one or more of the factors associated with CTDs—your best efforts may not prevent CTDs. My own experience is testimony to this fact.

In 1987, while writing a book on computer health and safety that discussed CTDs, I developed carpal tunnel syndrome. Even though I knew better, I set up my computer with the keyboard too high. When I typed, I had to bend my wrists sharply toward my palms—a position called flexion. As a risk factor, this would be classified as an *awkward position*. Because I happen to type rapidly and because writing a book requires long hours of work with few interruptions, I added two more risk factors, *high repetition rates* and *static postures*. A fourth factor in my case was that at that time I really pounded the keyboard, using a *high level of force*. I knew that this situation was potentially hazardous, but still did not recognize the symptoms of carpal tunnel syndrome when I first started waking up in the middle of night with hands that felt like buzzing lead weights.

When I did finally heed my symptoms, I was fortunate to be able to rearrange my work so that I could recover. For about one year I rarely touched a computer. That prolonged rest gave me that time I needed to heal so that I no longer felt pain. I also benefited enormously from studying a movement method called the Alexander Technique, a way of learning to use your body without unnecessary effort and tension. From this I learned how not to pound my keyboard.

Still, my hands now seem noticeably clumsier than they were before I developed carpal tunnel syndrome. Doctors tell me this is because I have lost some of the sensation in my hand and not because I actually have lost agility. I also have developed De Quervain's disease, which has weakened the thumb of my right hand. I used to open jars for my wife; now she opens them for me.

In 1992, during several months of intensive computer work, I developed tendinitis in my right forearm. I first tried a week of complete rest, but the pain returned as soon as I went back to my computer. Through exercise, a new computer desk that lowered my keyboard, and use of a track ball for input rather than a mouse, I gradually recovered.

How can someone knowledgeable about CTDs fall prey—twice? First, my work involves a high-risk activity, computer use. Second, I made matters worse by spending much too much time working at my computer.

My knowledge has paid off, nonetheless, enabling me to recognize telltale symptoms and to take pre-

ventive action. If I, like millions of American workers, had known very little about CTDs, I probably
would have accomplished a lot less over the past several years (an alarming thought for someone who is
self-employed) and suffered a lot more pain. In fact, I
probably would not have been able to write this book.

Mark A. Pinsky
Lower Makefield, PA

CHAPTER 1

Life with CTDs

In 1988, while working as an editor at the University of California at Berkeley, Joan Lichterman first noticed the symptoms that led to a diagnosis of carpal tunnel syndrome and related disorders in both of her hands and arms. She would wake at night with aching, tingling hands. Soon the tingling occurred at all hours. Her grip weakened and even simple things like carrying an umbrella and opening jars became difficult. Her hands often seemed tired. She found it increasingly difficult and painful to use her computer. Soon she could not hold a pen or pencil for more than a few minutes. Despite surgery in 1989, even simple things such as vacuuming her house were impossible.

"In the beginning, I couldn't even bathe myself very well," she says. "I couldn't put a bra on by myself. I learned to live with a lot more dirt and chaos in my immediate environment than I was used to."

In May 1992, presenting testimony to a U.S. Senate Labor Committee hearing on occupational safety and health, Lichterman reported that her condition had improved only slightly: "Although I am not in the acute pain I experienced earlier, I am not much better off than I was."

In the approximately three years since she was initially diagnosed with carpal tunnel syndrome, she had undergone two operations to release the pressure in her wrist, had taken anti-inflammatory medication for almost the entire time, and had put in hundreds of hours in physical and occupational therapy. During that period, she spent one year on disability leave from her job, eight months working half time, and another month and a half on disability. She had consulted "more physicians than anyone would ever care to see" and undergone physical therapy for movement reeducation and pain management.

Her diagnosis comprised carpal tunnel syndrome and "a whole range" of other disorders, too many for her to remember them all. She is still extremely limited and can do only a little for a very short time. She told the committee that to clean her bathtub she sprinkles it with cleanser, lets the cleanser sit for a while, and uses her feet to scrub the tub. "If I were to put such pressure on my hands they would be out of commission for a week. Other chores, such as washing the floors, are totally beyond me. My limit driving a car, even with [wrist] splints, is usually one hour a day, making it difficult to visit some friends or see a performance without a chauffeur. If I have done too much in a day, brushing my teeth sends shooting pains up my arms."

For four years, Lichterman believed that carpal tunnel syndrome was her primary health problem. It resulted, she believed, from long periods of work at her computer keyboard. The repetitive actions of typing, or keying, had caused swelling that pressed on the median nerve as it passed through the carpal tunnel, a small opening in the wrist surrounded on three sides by the eight carpal bones and on the palmar, or palm, side by the carpal ligament (*carpal* is Latin for "wrist").

In late 1992 she received new information that raised the possibility that she had been initially misdiagnosed. A doctor she consulted informed her that her carpal tunnel syndrome may have developed in part as a result of thoracic outlet syndrome. This condition is caused by compression, at the shoulder, of the brachial plexus, which includes the three main nerves that provide sensations to the arm and hand as well as the arteries and veins going to and from the arm.

From the onset of her illness in 1988, Lichterman had reported symptoms that made thoracic outlet syndrome a possible diagnosis. Her doctor at the time did not follow up on these symptoms and so did not order tests that might have clarified the diagnosis. Because Lichterman's symptoms did not clearly point to a case of carpal tunnel syndrome, the doctor took a wait-and-see approach and sent her back to work. "I accepted that 'doctor knows best' and went into a denial mode instead of seeking a second opinion," she remembers. "If anything, I worked on the computer even more intensively that next year, until the pain became disabling." Only then did the doctor diagnose her with carpal tunnel syndrome, a conclusion that appears to have been incomplete, if not incorrect.

The difficulty in getting an accurate diagnosis results from several factors: Many doctors are not trained to identify cumulative trauma disorders (CTDs), CTDs in their early stages are difficult to diagnose (medical tests are not always reliable even for advanced cases), there seems to be a high rate of multiple CTDs occurring simultaneously, and patients often fail to report their CTD symptoms thoroughly, assuming some of the symptoms are due to age or some other factor.

Now Lichterman wonders whether her doctor and therapists were treating the wrong problem and whether some of the treatment she received may have been doing her more harm than good. She concedes with a mix of anger and resignation that she made the mistake of not being aggressive about getting more tests done when she first reported her symptoms to her physician.

Today, Lichterman is passive no longer. Like a growing number of people with CTDs, she has channeled her frustration and anger into action. "Anger is empowering," she says. "If you can channel your anger in a constructive way, it really helps enormously.

Because you just can't feel helpless all the time and still live."

It may come as a surprise to learn that Lichterman considers herself one of the "lucky" permanently injured workers. The impact of her disability on other aspects of her life is, relatively speaking, limited. While her employer helped her return to work, other disabled CTD suffers have lost their homes because they could find no work that did not require use of their hands. Because she is single and childless, Lichterman is spared the feeling that she is not doing her share for her family. She has creatively negotiated with friends and others to barter her editing skills and computer knowledge for housecleaning and other help.

The physical pain and limitations "seem almost petty compared to the terror I have experienced." Like every other worker with serious CTDs, she worries about the future. "How can I support myself if my condition never improves? What will happen if my office is axed after the next round of budget cuts?" She has thought of returning to school for a teaching certificate but does not know how she would take notes and write papers. The Americans with Disability Act may prove to be a boon to people with CTDs, but it is as yet untested. "Do I have to sue a prospective employer, testing the limits of the new law, and wait at least a few years for an uncertain outcome?" Lichterman asks.

For many CTD sufferers, the emotional toll is great. "It just takes your dignity away when you can't take care of yourself," explains a former journalist. "I've lost who I was." Several people have felt such despair over the loss of their hands, and the resulting loss of their ability to contribute at home and to produce at work, that they considered suicide. "You have to try to make the best of it," Lichterman insists. "The alternative is to just be depressed all the time. You can't do it. It's no way to live."

Still, Lichterman cries when she talks about her own sense of loss. "When you can't use your hands you really lose the sense that you have any control over your life. I did a lot of wallowing for more than a year after I had surgery," she says. Particularly hard for her is the fact that she can no longer do crafts projects. "Around Christmas of 1989, a couple of months after I had the first surgery, I was still in nearly constant physical pain. While out on a walk to counter depression, I passed several craft shops and suddenly burst into tears. I returned home and sobbed for hours, thinking I'm never going to do this again.

"I am a craftsperson, and I don't know when I'll do crafts again. Or if I'll do them. There isn't going to be a miracle cure. It's too late," she says.

Carpal tunnel syndrome involves damage to the nerve going to the thumb and the three adjoining fingers. Compression can occur for many reasons ranging from a blow to your wrist to inflammation of your tendons. If identified early, carpal tunnel syndrome can be controlled and the damage limited. Untreated, it can advance quickly and cause permanent, and sometimes debilitating, injury. At its worst, it causes the loss of all functional use of the hands.

It is perhaps the most serious, though not the most common, of the array of upper extremity CTDs (sometimes referred to as repetition strain injuries, repetitive strain injuries, or repetitive motion injuries). The range of CTDs discussed in this book can be categorized as follows:

• *CTDs involving nerves*: carpal tunnel syndrome, thoracic outlet syndrome, ulnar nerve compression at the elbow, and ulnar nerve compression at the wrist.

• *CTDs involving tendons, muscles, and soft tissues*: bursitis, myositis, rotator cuff tendinitis, tendinitis (including tennis elbow and golfer's elbow), and tenosynovitis (including ganglion cysts, De Quervain's disease, and trigger finger).

• *CTDs involving the vascular (blood vessel) system*: Raynaud's syndrome and thoracic outlet syndrome.

Table 1.1 is a simple reference chart that you can use to learn more about the most common CTDs. Refer to Chapter 7 for more complete information.

Since 1981, there has been an alarmingly steep increase in the number of new work-related CTD cases. That number has skyrocketed from 18 percent of all reported on-the-job illnesses in 1981 to more than 60 percent, or about 223,600 workers, in 1991, according

Table 1.1 CTDs & Their Symptoms

Illness	Other Names	Primary Area Affected
Bursitis *See page 173*		Shoulder, elbow
Carpal tunnel syndrome *See page 174*	CTS, writer's cramp, occupational neuritis, partial thenar atrophy, median neuritis	Wrist and hand
Ganglion cyst *See page 189*	Bible bump	Wrist
Golfer's elbow (Medial epicondylitis) *See page 184*	Tendinitis	Inside of the elbow
Myositis *See page 184*	Muscle inflammation	Arm
Raynaud's syndrome *See page 185*	Raynaud's phenomenon, Raynaud's disease, Vibration syndrome	Hands and fingers
Rotator cuff tendinitis *See page 187*	Superspinatus, tendinitis, subdeltoid bursitis, subacromial bursitis, partial tear of the rotator cuff	Shoulder
Tennis elbow (Lateral epicondylitis) *See page 183*	Tendinitis, bowler's elbow, pitcher's elbow	Outside of the elbow
Tenosynovitis *See page 188*	Tendosynovitis, tendovaginitis, tenovaginitis, peritendinitis	Any tendon

Type	Symptoms
Connective tissue	(1) Grinding sensation. (2) Pain or irritation. (3) Restricted motion.
Nerve	(1) Tingling, pain, or numbness in the area of the hand served by the median nerve—the thumb, the pointing finger, the middle finger, and the half of the ring finger closest to the middle finger. Sensations also occur in the palm and back of the hand. In more advanced CTS, the pain can be excruciating. Symptoms often are more severe during sleep. (2) Loss of sensation, notably a feeling of clumsiness and loss of sensitivity to hot and cold.
Connective tissue	Bump or concentrated swelling.
Connective tissue	Pain or irritation on the inside of the elbow, often radiating down the arm.
Muscle	Aching, tiredness.
Vascular	(1) Unusual sensitivity to cold. (2) Pale, white, or blue hands, particularly following exposure to cold. (3) Occasional tingling or numbness. Can lead to loss on sensation and control.
Connective tissue	Pain, sometimes intense, or irritation in the shoulder.
Connective tissue	Pain or irritation on the outside of the elbow, often radiating down the forearm.
Connective tissue	(1) Pain or irritation, particularly while using the hand or arm. (2) Swelling can occur.

(continued)

Table 1.1 CTDs & Their Symptoms (*continued*)

Illness	Other Names	Primary Area Affected
Stenosing tenosynovitis *See page 189*		Any tendon
De Quervain's Disease *See page 189*	De Quervain's syndrome, De Quervain's disorder	Side and base of thumb
Trigger finger *See page 191*	Stenosing tenosynovitis crepitans	Forearm
Tendinitis *See page 186*	Tendonitis	Forearm, elbow, shoulder
Thoracic outlet syndrome *See page 191*	Neurovascular compression syndrome, hyperabduction syndrome, cervicobrachial disorder, brachial plexus neuritis, costoclavicular syndrome.	Shoulder, arm, hand
Ulnar nerve compression at the elbow *See page 193*	Cubital tunnel syndrome, cubital outlet syndrome, cubital canal syndrome, beer drinker's arm, telephone operator's arm	Elbow, forearm, hands
Ulnar nerve entrapment at the wrist *See page 194*	Guyon's canal syndrome, Guyon's tunnel syndrome	Wrist and Hand

Type	Symptoms
Connective tissue	(1) Pain or irritation. (2) Can result in uneven movement of fingers (see trigger finger).
Connective tissue	(1) Aching in affected area. (2) Weakness in thumb. (3) Loss of muscle tone (muscle atrophy).
Connective tissue	(1) Pain in the forearm or wrist. (2) Snapping or jerking movement of one or more fingers. (3) Rattling or crackling sound in hands or wrists.
Connective tissue	Pain or irritation, particularly while using the hand or arm.
Neurovascular	(1) Tingling and/or numbness in the fingers and hands. (2) Weak hands. (3) Atrophying muscles in the hand. (4) Pale or bluish hands (as in Raynaud's syndrome). (5) Arm pain. (6) Chronic tired arms.
Nerve	(1) Tingling, pain, or numbness in the area served by the ulnar nerve, particularly the little finger and the half of the ring finger closest to the little finger, as well as on the ulnar side of the hand and forearm. (The ulnar side is where the little finger is.) The sensation can be more severe at night. (2) Hand weakness.
Nerve	Decreased hand strength.

to the federal Bureau of Labor Statistics.* Even these figures are widely believed to underestimate the actual occurrence—perhaps by as much as 100 times—because of the way data are collected.

Jobs such as meat cutting, poultry processing, assembly line work, and production sewing have long been linked to arm and hand CTDs. Working with computers has more recently been added to that list (see Table 1-2). What these jobs share in common, and what research suggests are the primary factors linked to these ailments, are repetition, use of force, awkward postures, direct pressure, vibration, and prolonged work without postural changes. Psychosocial factors are now being added to the list, particularly for office work involving computers.

Indeed, the explosion of computer use since 1980 is one often-cited reason for the sharp rise in the number of cases, but it is only part of the picture. Vern Putz-Anderson of the National Institute for Occupational Safety and Health (NIOSH) has provided a broader explanation that accounts for the rise in CTD cases across blue-collar as well as white-collar occupations: "Automation has been successful in shifting the locus of work from the level of the trunk to the upper extremities [arms]. The workloads are now lighter, but the work pace has been increased. As a result, the as-

---

*The BLS maintains and publishes data on occupational illnesses and injuries in private industry. It treats ailments that were caused by a single incident, such as falling off a ladder, as *injuries*, while those resulting from chronic or cumulative causes are *illnesses*.

sociated work forces are concentrated on smaller parts
of the anatomy, i.e., the ligaments, tendons, muscles,
and nerves that control the hands, wrists, and arms of
a worker," he wrote in a 1988 article.

TABLE 1.2 Jobs Commonly Associated with CTDs

Assembly line workers
Buffers and grinders
Butchers
Carpenters
Computer operators
Electronic assemblers
Garment workers
Grocery checkers and cashiers
Janitors
Meat cutters
Musicians
Operating room personnel
Painters (house and industrial)
Postal carriers
Postal sorting clerks
Poultry processors
Punch press operators
Production sewers and seamstresses
Truck drivers
Typists

Joan Lichterman's experience is not uncommon
among people with carpal tunnel syndrome and other

CTDs. She had been disabled by the illness, and she has felt frustration and anger about the way she was treated in the workers' compensation system.

In at least four ways, however, her life after developing CTDs is markedly different from those of almost all other CTD sufferers.

• First, her employer went to unusual expense to accommodate her condition by installing an expensive voice-driven system that allowed her to continue to work at a computer. Until recently, the majority of workers with CTDs have had to fit themselves to the job and the working conditions. That is starting to change, at least in part due to the Americans with Disabilities Act of 1990, but the change is slow.

• Second, she started a support group, one of a loosely organized network of CTD support groups active in the San Francisco Bay area that has provided information on how to deal with CTDs, treatment and vocational options, and the workers' compensation system. Most people with CTDs are unaware of how common the condition is and never seek out others to discuss their problems and share their solutions.

One man who has had CTS surgery three times and is still in considerable pain has been trying to get his co-workers to consult their doctors before their conditions deteriorate. "I really don't think they've stopped and thought about it the way I have," he explains. "The one outstanding thing I've uncovered is there's a lot of ignorance out there about what they have and how they contracted the illness."

• Third, Lichterman has used her experience to press the federal government to step up its effort to combat the epidemic of job-related CTDs. "I wish I had more time to try to prevent people from having to go through this," she says. "That's one of the things that fuels me."

The Occupational Safety and Health Administration (OSHA), within the U.S. Department of Labor, has been talking about developing regulations to reduce job-related CTDs for years, but the agency has yet to decide whether to even propose a standard. In 1992, OSHA rejected a petition by a coalition of 31 labor unions for an "emergency" standard. The unions argued that the steep rise in the number of reported CTD cases represented a "grave danger" that merited extraordinary action. "Remedial measures to prevent these crippling disorders are known and well established," the unions reasoned. Lichterman warns that "OSHA can drag its feet for another twenty years unless they're forced to do something."

• Finally, she has had her say at two congressional hearings. On March 28, 1991, Lichterman testified before a House subcommittee chaired by Representative Tom Lantos. "We must make preventing repetitive strain injuries a priority, because I don't know of any cure," she argued. Little more than a year later, on May 6, 1992, she appeared before a Senate Labor Committee hearing. Introducing her, Committee

Chairman Senator Ted Kennedy said, "We will hear from Joan Lichterman, who has lost virtually all use of her hands from a syndrome that OSHA has refused to address."

Joan Lichterman is a token of hope, a reminder that by increasing awareness of CTD risk factors on the job, by providing healthy working conditions, by improving doctors' training, by informing people with CTDs about proper care, and by implementing an active federal campaign to control CTDs, we can sharply reduce their occurrence.

Many cases of carpal tunnel syndrome and other CTDs can be prevented or successfully treated if workers, employers, and doctors are better informed about their symptoms and causes, as well as about the options available for making jobs safer. That is both the most discouraging *and* the most encouraging fact about CTDs. It is discouraging because the lack of knowledge among workers and managers has resulted in harm to hundreds of thousands of people over the past decade alone and hundreds of millions of dollars in medical and other costs to people with CTDs, their employers, and insurance companies.

Training for doctors in treating CTDs is inadequate in many instances, as well. *Business Week* magazine, in a 1989 editorial, brusquely challenged both employers and physicians to sit up and take notice. "Although repetitive motion injuries have been known for many years, many doctor still don't realize that the problem can stem from the workplace," the editorial charged. It closed with an equally harsh criticism of business owners: "If employers don't want an epidemic of these injuries, they must face up to the dangerous workplace potential of new technology." Such a strong stand from a magazine that is plainly probusiness clearly reflects the need to take CTDs seriously. By 1993, there were only a few faint signs that business had heeded this advice.

For business, there is an economic reason, as well as a compassionate one, to address the CTD epidemic aggressively. Estimates place the cost of CTDs on private sector American businesses at more than $25 billion per year in workers' compensation and disability insurance, lost work time, and decreased productivity. Not included in these estimates are potential liability costs in the hundreds of millions or more for companies that produce equipment, such as computer keyboards, that are being blamed for CTDs. And in federal, state, and local government workers—the U.S. Postal Service consistently has had some of the highest rates of CTDs in the world—and the potential costs to the economy reach even higher.

The encouraging aspect about finding ways to prevent CTDs is that a little knowledge in the workplace and in the doctor's office will go a long way. Better awareness and understanding of the problem is the best solution for long-term, productivity-enhancing results, explains Dr. Steven Barrer, a neurosurgeon in Abington, Pennsylvania, who specializes in carpal tunnel syndrome. Writing in the January 1991 issue of *Occupational Health & Safety* magazine, Barrer states, "Clearly, what's needed is a multi-faceted program of education, prevention, and treatment."

CHAPTER 2

What Causes CTDs?

If you or your doctor believe that you have developed a CTD, you should try to figure out what caused it. What have you done in your work, your hobbies, or at other times that might be CTD-related? If you are a meat cutter, a computer data entry clerk, or a violinist, the answer may be apparent.

For others, the answer may be more difficult to pin down. There are several known and possible causes of carpal tunnel syndrome and other CTDs. Each can produce a CTD alone or in combination with other factors.

If your work involves more than one CTD risk factor, the combination "markedly increases" the chances that you will develop a CTD, warns Dr. David Rempel of the University of California at San Francisco's Division of Occupational Medicine. Overlooking a factor can also prevent you from addressing the whole problem.

By definition CTDs develop over time rather than as the result of a single incident. Your illness could have started in a job you held several years ago. For it to have reached a stage where you notice the symptoms, however, there must still be something that is contributing to the disorder.

The factors most specialists agree are associated with CTDs of the arm and hand are:

- Repetition

- High force

- Awkward postures

- Direct pressure

- Vibration

- Unvarying work positions.

Some researchers also add stress-related factors to this list—so-called psychosocial issues such as control over your work flow, relations with your co-workers and with your supervisor, and your day-to-day authority to make decisions.

This chapter will help you to identify risk factors in your job. Without having to learn a lot of engineering and industrial design terms, you can evaluate your working conditions to reduce the risk of developing a CTD. If you already have a work-related disorder, you can identify possible causes so that you can make your work place safer for yourself and your co-workers.

Approach this task with an open mind. Don't fixate on one apparent cause to the exclusion of others. For example, while your job may involve a lot of repetition, do not overlook the pace or the work posture. You may need to experiment with a variety of potential solutions before you successfully address the causes of your problem.

In addition, there is scientific uncertainty about how closely to link some risk factors to CTDs. The uncertainty is not so much whether the identified factors are real concerns as it is which factors pose the greatest risk and what combinations are most hazardous. There simply are not enough research data to draw these conclusions, says Dr. Lawrence Fine of NIOSH.

You may not be able to make all of the changes you believe are needed because your supervisor or employer is not convinced your analysis is correct. He or she may resist making changes in work practices or purchasing new equipment. Be as thorough as possible in documenting your symptoms and the risk factors in your job. It will be up to you, and possibly your co-workers, to negotiate any changes with your employer.

Table 2.1 summarizes risk factors that have been associated with a variety of jobs and shows which CTDs appear to be most common for workers in those jobs. (If you need help understanding some of the

Table 2.1
Selected Work Activities, Risk Factors, and CTDs

Job	Risk Factors
Assembly line work	Repeated, forceful wrist motions, Extreme extension, abduction, or flexion of arms and/or wrists
Buffing and grinding	Repeated wrist motions, prolonged shoulder flexion, Vibration, Forceful ulnar deviation, Repeated forearm pronation
Carrying a mail bag	Prolonged heavy load on shoulder, Repeated shoulder abduction and adduction
Cleaning and scrubbing	Repeated ulnar and radial wrist deviation, repeated hand flexion and extension
Computer keying	Prolonged postures, rapid finger movements with wrists flexed or extended, ulnar deviation
Driving a truck/bus/car	Prolonged shoulder abduction and flexion, Prolonged gripping
Meat cutting and poultry processing	Repeated ulnar deviation, repeated wrist flexion with exertion
Playing music (some instruments)	Repeated wrist motions, prolonged shoulder abduction and flexion, forceful wrist extension, forceful forearm pronation
Sewing and cutting	Repeated shoulder flexion, repeated ulnar deviation, repeated wrist flexion and extension, pressure on the base of the palm, stress
Supermarket checking	Repeated ulnar deviation, repeated shoulder abduction and adduction
Small parts assembling	Prolonged restrictive posture, forceful ulnar deviations and thumb pressure, repeated wrist motion, forceful wrist extension and pronation
Working overhead (welding, painting, repairing cars)	Repeated ulnar deviation, sustained hyperextension of arms, hands above shoulders

Commonly Associated CTDs

Tendinitis in the wrist and shoulder (rotator cuff), tenosynovitis, carpal tunnel syndrome, thoracic outlet syndrome

Tenosynovitis, thoracic outlet syndrome, carpal tunnel syndrome, De Quervain's disease

Rotator cuff tendinitis, thoracic outlet syndrome

Tendinitis, carpal tunnel syndrome, De Quervain's disease

Tendinitis, tenosynovitis, carpal tunnel syndrome, De Quervain's disease, ulnar nerve entrapment at the wrist

Thoracic outlet syndrome, carpal tunnel syndrome, tendinitis

Carpal tunnel syndrome, tendinitis in the wrist, tenosynovitis in the wrist, De Quervain's disease

Tendinitis in the wrist, carpal tunnel syndrome, tennis elbow

Thoracic outlet syndrome, carpal tunnel syndrome, De Quervain's disease

Carpal tunnel syndrome, tendinitis in the wrist and shoulder, thoracic outlet syndrome

Thoracic outlet syndrome, tendinitis in the wrist, tennis elbow

Tendinitis in the wrist and shoulder (rotator cuff), carpal tunnel syndrome, ganglion cyst, thoracic outlet syndrome terms in the table, refer to the glossary in the back of this book.)

There are four main areas to analyze for possible CTD causes in your job:

• *The physical working environment.* No matter what type of job you do, you should have equipment, tools, and working conditions that are appropriate to the work and to you. If you feel comfortable in your chair when you start the day but uncomfortable by lunch, that's a clear sign that you need to make changes.

• *The movements the job requires.* Your job may require unusual exertion, repetition, or postures. Even if this does not *seem* to describe your work, evaluate your job carefully. Working with your elbows resting on a workbench all day may seem normal, but could it be the reason your hands tingle and feel weaker than they used to?

• *The social working environment.* Computer pacing and automation can create stressful working conditions, but so can piecework. Many other aspects of your job can produce stress (such as an overbearing supervisor or an underproductive staff). Are you aware of them all?

• *The way you do the movements and respond to the social environment.* Everyone is different. Some people are naturally more tense—physically and emotionally—than others. Could you learn new ways of responding to the demands of your work that might help prevent CTDs?

Your Physical Working Environment

Most of us take our working conditions for granted. You are happy to have your own desk . . . it never occurred to you that it might not be the right height for your computer keyboard. You enjoy working with your hands and you have all the tools you need . . . you probably never noticed that you hunch over your work station all day because the light is too dim.

Try to take a step back from your working environment so that you can see it with fresh eyes. Following are some things you might look for:

Work Surface Height

For an auto mechanic, the work surface is often a foot or two above his head. For a computer operator, the keyboard should be between 21 inches and 23 inches above the floor.

There is no such thing as one "proper" height since jobs vary so widely. You want a work surface that allows you to do your job without unusual strain. If your job is to pack books into boxes and the empty box is on a shelf two feet in front of your at shoulder level, you will strain your arms every time you reach inside the box. In addition, you will have to bend your wrists and may have to position your elbows at awkward angles.

The work surface should be just below elbow height when you are in your normal working position (sitting or standing) and within two feet of your torso so that you can reach it without contorting or straining your body. A work surface that is too high forces you to lift your arms and hold them away from your body. One that is too low forces you to bend over and to reach with your hands, often in awkward positions.

Auto mechanics, carpenters, and others who use power hand tools should take particular care to adjust the heights of their work surfaces so that the elbow of the hand holding the tool is approximately at a right angle. Power tools add vibration, another CTD risk factor, to your working condition (see page 34).

If you sit while you work, the surface should be comfortably above your thighs but only high enough that you can do your job with your wrists in a neutral position (neither flexed nor extended).

Seating

Chair seats and backs should be wide enough to support all of you. A properly designed chair supports your back, legs, and torso and indirectly supports your head, neck, and arms. It is a stable base from which you can comfortably and confidently do even the most delicate work. A stool may be acceptable if you sit for brief, intermittent periods. But every person

who spends most of the working time seated should
have a chair with:

• A *back support* that presses firmly against at least
the lower half of your back. Old-fashioned secretary
chairs with narrow back supports are inadequate for
prolonged sitting.

• A *seat* that easily adjusts to tilt backward and forward and that supports your thighs almost to your
knees but not so far that you cannot sit with your legs
comfortably bent. It must be wide enough that you do
not feel as if you are sliding off.

• *A one-lever adjustment for height*. Many chair
manufacturers promote their products' ergonomic fea-
tures, but you need a chair that adjusts *easily*. This is
particularly important if you share you chair with a
co-worker.

When your chair is adjusted properly, your feet
should rest comfortably on the ground. Some people
may need a footrest.

Too many companies purchase ergonomically correct chairs but then tell their workers not to adjust
them for proper fit. Dr. Marvin Dainoff, an ergonomist who specializes in office chairs and computer
work stations, says one company executive called to
complain about the new chairs Dainoff had recommended. Dainoff found all the chairs still set to their
lowest heights, just as they had come out of their ship-
ping boxes. The supervisor thought that the chairs had

been precisely calibrated at the factory and that he shouldn't mess with them. "Meanwhile, his people were working in completely inappropriate positions," Dainoff says.

Direct Pressure

Beware of sharp edges and other surfaces that can put pressure directly on your arms and hands while you work. Postal carriers often cannot avoid direct pressure on their shoulders, but assembly line workers should not have to reach over or around a sharp corner to do their jobs.

Lighting

Lighting is not an obvious thing to consider when you are concerned about your arms and hands. But there are two aspects of lighting in your workplace that you should evaluate:

• *Is the lighting sufficient?* When there is not enough light for you to see what you are doing at a safe working height, you have two choices—you can bend over to get closer to your work or you can bring your work closer to your eyes.

In the first case you put too much pressure on your back, and you also are likely to hunch your shoulders and force your arms and possibly your hands into awkward positions. This is unacceptable. In the second case, your arms have to work all day to hold an object up off of the work surface that was designed to support it. This strains the muscles and tendons.

• *Is glare hindering your work?* Glare is a major concern for computer users, since unwanted light can make it difficult to read their computer screens. Unless the glare problem is fixed, computer users will find themselves leaning from side to side or stretching up and hunching down in their seats to get a good viewing angle. This is certain to put their arms and hands in awkward positions.

Glare can also be an issue in factories and other settings where computers are not in use. If you find yourself shifting around at your workstation to avoid glare, it is easy to look around for the source of the problem.

Keyboards and Other Computer Equipment

Computer keyboards—and how they are used—are often associated with CTDs. Every day, millions of people work all day doing little else than typing away at the keys. The fastest typists can press more than 13,000 keys in an hour. Several factors can increase the risk associated with repetition:

• *Height.* If the keyboard is too high or too low, your arms and hands are forced into awkward positions. Your wrists will be either flexed (for a keyboard that is too high) or extended (for one that is too low), putting pressure on your tendons and your median nerves.

• *Tilt*. Almost all new keyboards come with adjustable legs that allow you to adjust the tilt. Most are designed to tilt with the back edge (nearest the computer) higher than the front edge, but some computer health specialists believe that keyboards tilted the other direction—the back edge lower than the front, or back-tilted—do a better job of keeping your wrists in a neutral position. If you are working with a back-tilted keyboard, it is crucial that the keyboard not be too high, since this will force you to flex your wrists sharply (bend them toward your palms) and also will force your arms into awkward positions.

• *Wrist rests*. If your keyboard drops off sharply in the front, you may find yourself extending your wrists (bending toward the back of your hands). This strains your muscles and tendons. It also can cause compression of the median nerves, a condition that can lead to carpal tunnel syndrome. There is a wide selection of wrist rests you can use to help prevent this from happening.

• *Keying pressure*. If you work at a keyboard with keys that are hard to press down, your hands probably tire rapidly. This type of keyboard requires extra force. When you are pressing as many as 13,000 keys an hour, a "hard" keyboard can increase your risk of developing a CTD.

At the opposite extreme, an overly sensitive, or soft, keyboard can lead you to constantly hold your hands above the keyboard for fear that a single brush of a key could show up as a character on screen. This means that you steadily contract the muscles on the back side of your forearms to keep your wrists slightly extended so that your fingers do not drop on the keys. In addition, you will soon be pulling up at the shoulder joint to suspend your arms.

• *Keyboard layout.* There should be sufficient space among the keys to allow your fingers to find the right key comfortably. Most new keyboards are spacious, but if you use a portable computer you may find that the keys are close together. If you keep your fingers unnaturally close together while you type, the keyboard may be the cause.

Portable computers with small keyboards also exaggerate a condition caused by most standard keyboards—you have to bend your wrists toward your little fingers (ulnar deviation). A new generation of keyboards addresses this problem. These keyboards are split in the middle (approximately between the "6" key and the "7" key) and the parts can be rotated to reduce ulnar deviation (for more on these keyboards, see Chapter 3).

• *Tools.* A screwdriver is a screwdriver is a screwdriver. Or is it? Electricians who use screwdrivers all day know the difference between one with a small, plastic handle and another one with a larger, rubber-coated handle.

Every tool, from an old-fashioned screwdriver to a cordless drill to a pneumatic bolt fastener, can affect your health.

• *Handle size and shape*. A handle that is too small makes you grasp it with your fingers rather than with your entire hand. This puts an extra work load on the muscles in your forehand simply to hold the tool, and can add considerable strain when you use the tool. Instead of using your entire arm and body to turn a small-handled screwdriver, for example, you must primarily use just your forearm muscles.

An oversized handle also imbalances the distribution of work. You are forced to use the large muscles in your upper arm, limiting the agility gained from your forearm muscles.

Pliers and other grip tools that have sharp edges can press on the tendons in the palms of your hands and irritate them. Look for tools with rounded edges and rubber-coated handles.

• *Handle Angle*. Pliers give you a good idea of the need for different handle angles for different jobs. A plumber trying to reach pipes under a sink, for example, will have an easier job if he has several pliers that bend at different angles.

Handle angles can be just as important for other tools. If you work on an assembly line tightening bolts with a power bolt driver, the tool's handle should allow you to reach the bolts without lifting your entire arm up elbow first so that you can put the tool on to the bolts. This also can force you to bend your wrist sharply in the direction of your little finger or your thumb. Doing this thousands of times daily could prove hazardous.

In some instances, you may need to change your work surface height as well as the tool handle.

• *Electronic controls.* A punch press operator may press an electronic control thousands of times a day. The control should be within easy reach. These controls commonly were located overhead for many years, requiring the operator to reach up. Newer designs place the control at about waist level, sometimes even allowing it to be moved for comfort and safety.

• *Proper maintenance.* One of the most common— and most overlooked—problems in factories is tools that have lost their edge. If a ratchet wrench is not properly lubricated, you may have to work twice as hard as you should each time you pull the handle.

Consider a meat cutter with a dull knife. Not surprisingly, knives lose their sharpness rapidly in meat processing plants. Some meat processing companies have started adding knife-sharpening programs in the meat cutting area—sometimes even adding workers to sharpen knives—so that meat cutters will always have properly maintained tools.

Vibration

Equipment such as buffers, sanders, and jackhammers that vibrate constantly can put stress on the joints and muscles in your your arm and hand. In addition, vibration is known to cause blood vessels in the fingers to constrict. Over time, this can lead to Raynaud's syndrome. Use of these tools is further complicated by the tendency to hold them with an unusually firm grip, increasing the extent of the vibration transferred to the arm. Vibrating tools that involve repetitive motions, such as power sanding, have been associated with carpal tunnel syndrome.

Temperature

Working in a cold environment has been linked to CTDs. The generally accepted guideline is that a constant working temperature below 70 degrees can be considered a risk factor. Temperature is particularly important if one or more other factors also exist at your job.

The Movements You Make

Signing for the deaf does not seem to belong in the same category as building cars, but Jaspar Shealy says that when it comes to CTDs they are. "Signing is a lot like working on an assembly line," according to Shealy, who is chairman of the Department of Industrial and Manufacturing Engineering at the Rochester Institute of Technology (RIT) in New York.

Shealy has informally studied signers at RIT's National Technical Institute for the Deaf, and he hopes to undertake a large, long-term study of CTDs among signers. He has observed a "fairly high" rate of CTDs among the 70 full-time and 100 to 150 part-time signers associated with the institute. The types of movements that signers make with their fingers, hands, and arms can make the job hazardous, Shealy believes. About two years ago, before the signers were given hand warm-up exercises and told they could work no more than four hours a day, down from five, almost 20 percent were either on long-term disability insurance or had taken early retirement because of CTDs.

Repetitive motions, like other movement-related risk factors for CTDs, are not always obvious. This section explains key characteristics of the movements involved in many jobs so that you can begin to recognize potential problems in your work.

Repetition

"The human body was simply not made to perform thousands of repetitive motions an hour. The electronic revolution has outstripped our human muscular and skeletal evolution," warns Dr. Linda Morse of the Repetitive Motion Institute in San Jose, California.

Computerization and automation have made repetition the hallmark of modern jobs. Anyone who has stood in one place along an assembly line for eight

hours a day, day in and day out, knows that repetitive
work can be monotonous, tiring, and frustrating.

But modern assembly lines no longer allow as
much variety of movements as assembly lines once
did. It used to be that when you worked on an assembly line building a car, for example, you had to push
the parts along to the next station, giving you a break
from the repetitive task that made up your job. Now a
conveyor belt allows you to stay in one place, and
your job has been simplified to one or two tasks—
tightening bolts, for instance, or installing wind-
shields. While the older methods may have frustrated
both workers and management, the slower pace gave
muscles, tendons, and ligaments time to recover.

Every job involves repetitive motions, which can
pose a risk when they make up a significant share of
what you do during a day and when they are not offset
by sufficient rest and recovery periods. When your muscles contract rapidly and repeatedly, they operate with
less tension and every contraction takes more effort.
Greater effort requires greater recovery time. In repetitive jobs where the recovery periods are insufficient to
begin with, the situation can spiral out of control (see
Table 2.2).

Table 2.2 Repetition Rates for Selected Jobs

Assembly line work	Up to 25,000 movements daily
Computer keying	Up to 13,000 keys hourly
Poultry processing	Up to 15,120 cuts per day
Signing for the deaf	Up to 13,600 movements hourly
Sorting mail	Up to 23,000 motions daily

As easy as it is to think of computer data entry as the model of repetitive work, you may be subjecting yourself to at least as much repetition if your job is polishing cars with an electric, hand-held buffer. More important, the risk may be higher.

Jobs that involve both high repetition rates and the use of force merit special concern. In a 1987 study that analyzed whether repetition or force was a greater risk factor for carpal tunnel syndrome, Barbara Silverstein, Dr. Lawrence Fine, and Thomas Armstrong developed a scale for ranking whether specific jobs involved high or low repetition as well as high or low force.

They found that "repetitiveness appeared to be a stronger risk factor than force." They also found, however, that jobs that were both highly repetitious and involved high force were most clearly linked to carpal tunnel syndrome. "High force combined with high repetitiveness appears to have more than a multiplicative effect, increasing the risk more than five times that of either factor alone."

Force

It is easy to distinguish jobs requiring a lot of muscle force (i.e., lifting heavy objects) from those needing low levels (i.e., computer keying). It is primarily a question of how hard you have to work, physically, to do your job.

A wide range of factors affect how much force you use. Lifting an object requires more force if you do it in an *awkward position* than if you do it properly. A *slippery object* is harder to hold on to than is one that is easy to grip. The shape of the object will determine what kind of *grip* you can use—gripping with your fingertips is more likely to lead to CTDs than gripping with your whole hand. For example, it is easier to lift a heavy box that has handles than one you must grip from underneath.

Awkward postures

Most of us are so used to working in slightly awkward positions that we do not fully account for the hazards they can pose. You recognize that you could strain your elbow if you tried to pick up something heavy with your arm reaching too far away from your body. You may not be aware that your job puts you into similarly awkward situations every day.

Auto mechanics spend most of their work day with their arms above their heads or with their fingers and hands working with small parts in tight spaces. These are intrinsically awkward postures. The saving grace for mechanics may be that their jobs usually also involve chores such as retrieving parts, test driving cars, and other tasks that provide breaks from the awkward positions.

Do not overlook awkward postures in your job, particularly if they also involve repetition or force. They can cause you to misuse or overuse your joints, muscles, and tendons. Ultimately, posture determines how long you can perform your job without undue risk, warns Putz-Anderson.

In reviewing your work for awkward postures, you should also think about the physical characteristics of your workplace (see page 25). If your chair is difficult to adjust, your work surface is too high, or the lighting is wrong, the odds are good that you are compensating with awkward postures.

Try going through the motions of your work at home, mimicking the things you do most often. In particular, watch what you are doing with your joints:

• Are your wrist and hand regularly bending in one direction or another?

• Is your forearm twisting one way or the other?

• Are you pressing up against hard or sharp surfaces?

• Are your elbows or wrists resting on your work surface?

• Are your shoulders hunched or your arms pulled away from your body?

Grips

Your grip is strongest when your wrist is either in a neutral position (neither flexed nor extended) or slightly extended (bent toward the back of your hand). When your wrist is flexed (bent toward the palm) or bent sideways in either direction (ulnar deviation when it is bent toward the little finger and radial deviation when it is bent toward the thumb), your grip is weakened.

A *power grip* is what you use when you hold a hammer. It can become hazardous if you sustain it for long periods, make repetitive motions, or use high levels of force. Carpenters and meat cutters both are subject to this. In the meat cutting industry, one solution that has been tried is a bent-handle knife that eliminates the ulnar deviation of the wrist.

A *precision grip* uses the fingers, which get their strength from muscles in the forearm via tendons that travel through the wrist. This grip combined with repeated motions over long periods can produce CTDs. Assembling small parts such as electronic semiconductor boards on an assembly line involves repeated precision gripping. When force or awkward postures are added to tasks using precision grips, the risk increases. If the semiconductor boards are moving along an assembly line that is either too high or too low, the task of assembling them may well involve multiple hazards.

Unchanging Postures

Not moving enough can contribute to CTDs just as moving too much can. Unchanging, or static, postures require your muscles to sustain you in one position for loner than they are made to do. The muscles get tired quickly and transfer some of the work load to tendons and ligaments, making these tissues more vulnerable.

In addition, this type of muscle-holding—in contrast to muscles that are regularly contracting and elongating—amounts to a lack of exercise, making your body more susceptible to illness.

Your Social Working Environment

Not only where you work but who you work with, who you work for, how you get along with your coworkers and supervisor, and how your job is organized can affect your chances of developing a CTD. Even the economy can play a role if you feel that your job may be eliminated. While these and related psychosocial factors, as they are known, seem to play more of a role in CTDs in office work, where they have been studied more extensively, many also apply to all jobs.

The boom in computer use in offices has produced more social isolation, less worker control over jobs, and counterproductive steps in the areas of job security, work load, and work pace, according to Dr. Michael Smith of the University of Wisconsin at Madison. Smith's comments at a conference on video display terminal (VDT) health and safety in Berlin, Germany, in September 1992, reflect a shift in thinking on CTDs and computer use, according to *VDT News,* a newsletter reporting on health hazards associated with computer use. "Many [researchers] who came to Berlin argued that the nature of the job—not the choice of tools—is the most important issue," the newsletter reported.

Dr. Larry Fine of NIOSH says that research shows a significant difference between CTDs in offices and in traditionally blue-collar work settings. "In the blue collar, manufacturing, assembly line type of situation, the predominant factors are physical ones—force, repetition, awkward postures, and direct trauma to the hand. In office settings with keyboard use, focusing simply on the physical factors does not seem as productive as focusing on both the physical and psychosocial factors. Psychosocial factors seem to be more important," he says.

Fine's conclusions are based on more than 25 investigations NIOSH has done since 1979. Taken together, the investigations—Health Hazard Evaluations, they are called—represent one of the most informative sets of data on CTD causes and solutions available in the United States (see chapter 3).

One of the Health Hazard Evaluations may be crucial. The 1992 investigation found that production pressure and workers' concerns about job security and other psychosocial factors were consistent indicators of a CTD risk among computer users in the Denver, Minneapolis, and Phoenix offices of US West Communications. As many as one in five of these employees developed CTDs. About 15 percent of the workers had tendon-related disorders, 8 percent had muscle-related disorders, and 4 percent had nerve-entrapment disorders such as carpal tunnel syndrome. Some

Table 2.3

Psychosocial Variables Evaluated in the US West Health Hazard Evaluation

Boring work
Computer monitor quality
Computer monitors quantity
Control over amount and quality of work
Control over job-related matters
Control over work policy and materials
Cooperation between union and management
    on health issues
Customer hostility
Fear of being replaced by a computer
High information processing demands
Increasing work load
Increasing work pressure
Job requires a variety of tasks
Job satisfaction
Lack of co-worker support
Lack of friends' and relatives' support
Lack of supervisor support
Little interaction with others
Little interaction with co-workers
Meaningful work
Participation in work decisions
Presence of a productivity standard
Skill utilization
Sum of supervisor, co-worker, and home support
Sum of work load mental demands
Uncertainty about job future
Work requires high mental demands
Work requires very little thinking

workers had more than one CTD (see Table 2.3 for a

list of psychosocial factors considered in the US West study).

Before the study began, US West had significantly improved the physical working conditions in response to a high number of CTD cases. In addition, the company had taken notice of the decision by 30 ailing US West employees to file suit against a keyboard manufacturer. The company had also sued the manufacturer to recover the medical costs associated with the CTD epidemic. Both suits were settled out of court, and the terms of the settlements are secret.

VDT News reported that at the Berlin Conference, US West was cited repeatedly as a prime example of the limits of prevention strategies based only on physical ergonomics—and of the need for new ways to organize work schedules and reduce job stress. This was supported by a NIOSH investigation that found that while most workstations complied with current ergonomic guidelines, illness rates remained high.

Fine says the study seems to show that physical factors alone aren't important. From a practical perspective on CTDs, he says, you need to look at both the physical and psychosocial factors. As director of the Division of Surveillance, Hazard Evaluations, and Field Studies at NIOSH, Fine is responsible for all health hazard evaluations.

Fine confirmed the important role that psychosocial factors can play by reanalyzing the data from the US West evaluation in a follow-up study. Fine and others were concerned that the US West results could have occurred because workers with CTDs were more likely to complain about the stress-related problems than were healthy employees. Fine tested this point by studying CTD rates in relation to the psychosocial conditions reported by the *uninjured* workers. He found that the associations between CTDs and psychosocial conditions remained significant.

The evidence that psychosocial factors may cause or contribute to CTDs clearly needs follow-up, but Fine says there are two significant obstacles. The first is that people are more willing, and better able, to change physical factors. The second hurdle is that there is, and will probably continue to be, a research gap. No one has done the kind of study that needs to be done to give a reliable read on how psychosocial factors and physical ones interact in CTD cases, Fine explains. As one of the top federal officials overseeing occupational health research, he doesn't believe this kind of study will be done in the foreseeable future because of the high cost involved.

One of the best available models for understanding how psychosocial factors affect workers' health is Robert Karasek's simple matrix that plots jobs by two factors: the amount of latitude a worker has in decision making and the degree of psychological demand in a job (for instance, production pressure). Natural scientists and therapists, for example, have low job stress—lots of decision making discretion and little psychological pressure. On the other hand, industrial seamstresses, data entry clerks, telephone operators, and cashiers have little decision latitude and relatively high psychological demands, and so are considered high-stress occupations.

You can assess the social working environment in your job by weighing the following factors:

Management Styles

When there is a problem at work—anything from a failure to meet a production quota to the illness of your child—are you comfortable talking to your supervisor?

Every supervisor, manager, or business owner has a unique management method. Some encourage employees to suggest ways to improve working conditions, while others discourage them. At two U.S. Postal Service facilities, workers feared reporting symptoms of CTDs because there was a history of reprisals, according to a 1991 analysis prepared for the Occupational Safety and Health Administration (OSHA) by Dr. William Marras of Ohio State University. More than 90 percent of the workers in the study who had operated letter sorting machines said they had CTD symptoms, but the postal service's official OSHA logs reported a much lower rate.

Job Control

Who makes decisions for you moment by moment? If you make all decisions, you have a high degree of job control. If, to the contrary, you make no decisions because you do the same simple task over and over, then you have no job control.

The increasing automation and computerization of work through the 1980s has led to "deskilling." When a job is deskilled, it is stripped to its bare essentials. Where a secretary once would have typed letters, proofread the letters, and made corrections, all while answering phones, managing files, and greeting visitors, in many offices today there is a data entry pool, a proofreader, a phone message center (or voice mail), a filing clerk, and a visitor's center.

Not only has this taken discretion away from the secretary, it has also removed job variations. The job applicant who once might have been given a secretarial job now is likely to end up in the data entry pool, where he or she will do just one thing.

Deskilled jobs often are repetitive ones, making job control not merely a psychosocial concern for CTD risks but one with direct implications for the physical aspects of work, as well.

Pacing and Monitoring

One of the best known effects of automation and computerization is that the pace of work often is no longer controlled by the worker. This is not a new problem—many people laughingly recall what happened to Lucy Ricardo on the old *I Love Lucy* television series when a candy-making conveyor belt outpaced her ability to pack the finished candy pieces.

The addition of computers to automation created a new issue, however.

Since a computer can monitor not only how much a single worker produces but how many keystrokes she makes in a given period, pacing has achieved an unprecedented level of micromanagement. Workers are forced to perform at peak levels without sufficient rest. Computers can work at whatever speed is necessary, so worker performance is the limit to productivity increases. In many instances, the computers are set to work at a pace designed for the "average" worker. For many workers, the average pace is above their capacity.

In addition, research being done by Drs. Steven Sauter and Naomi Swanson at NIOSH suggests that uninterrupted peak performance does not produce the highest achievable output. In a study reported at the Berlin VDT conference, the scientists found that periodic mini-rest breaks and frequent, thirty-second "micropauses" in addition to regular breaks improved performance and lowered reports of discomfort among VDT operators. Sauter and Swanson noted that "even though the added breaks cut into the total amount of time workers were engaged in their data-entry task, their overall output for the day was higher than that of the workers who took less frequent breaks," according to *VDT News*.

If you are paid on the basis of piecework, as many seamstresses are, you are subject to another equally stressful form of pacing. The pressure to maximize production is great when your income is directly tied to how much you produce, particularly when no significant value is placed on the quality of the work.

Still another type of pacing is the "average work time" system used by some telephone service companies, including local phone companies and catalog phone-order services. The company management uses data gathered by measuring the amount of time a phone inquiry or order takes to set an average work time it can use to rate its workers. In some cases, workers' pay is linked to their performance relative to the average work time.

Perhaps you have had the experience while calling a telephone operator that he attempts to rush you off the line after about twenty or twenty-five seconds. This may have happened because his average work time—the amount of time in which he is expected to complete his job—is thirty seconds.

Job Security

Few things cause more anxiety than the thought that your job may be in jeopardy. During much of the 1980s, several things happened in the economy that made job security a thing of the past for many workers.

There was a steady decline in the number of blue-collar jobs, displacing millions of workers. The computerization of offices forced employees to undergo job retraining, much of it on the job. Computer-based monitoring gave managers a new way of rating employees. For some workers who were used to doing their jobs well, the shift to computers and to computer-based evaluations did not go smoothly.

The relative decline of the U.S. economy compared to that of foreign nations combined with the new-found ability to locate data entry jobs overseas (another result of computerization) meant there were fewer jobs to go around. Employers relied on overtime rather than hiring additional employees. Finally, employed workers who once might have switched jobs for advancement held on to their positions more tightly.

The result? Fewer jobs and a more competitive job market.

Several specialists cite this decrease in job security as a significant psychosocial factor relating to CTDs. "In times when there were plenty of jobs, people with sore hands probably left that job and went to another one," says NIOSH's Larry Fine. Now they stay in their jobs, concerned not only that they might lose their job, but also that doing their jobs might be harming them.

Relationships with Co-Workers

Stress can enter your work life not only from your relationship to your supervisor or employer, but also from your relationship to your co-workers. If you are in competition with a colleague for a promotion, or if you feel another person is getting preferential treatment for any reason, your work may seem unpleasant and stressful. You may not want to admit that your wrists or hands are ailing, because doing so might place you at a competitive disadvantage.

How You Make the Movements and Respond to the Social Environment

Arthur Georgantas, a sales representative for a major East Coast food cooperative, attributes his carpal tunnel syndrome to the way he held the steering wheel while driving, which he does extensively. He first identified three aspects of his job that involved repetition and so were suspect as possible causes of his illness—driving, writing, and stocking supermarket shelves. "The more I learn about carpal tunnel syndrome and just become aware of what I do, I've concluded that the one repetitive thing I do every day, day in and day out, is driving. I do that between three and five and a half hours daily."

He and others in the company persuaded their employer to hire a specialist in fitting equipment to people—a profession known as ergonomics—who they hope will help them understand how to prevent further problems. "You may be doing something incorrectly, but it's really just out of plain ignorance," he said. "In elementary school, they teach you how to sit when you write, but no one ever told me how to sit when I drive."

Training people how to use the tools and equipment they need for their work is often overlooked. No matter how well designed and easily adjustable a computer workstation is, it will not help reduce the incidence of CTDs if the people using it do not know how to fit it to their needs and why it's to their advantage to do so.

"You can't impose an ergonomic solution on your employees and expect the problem to go away," reasons Marvin Dainoff, who believes that you must not only show workers how to use equipment but that you must also involve them in the decision making that leads to installing it.

Dainoff also advocates ergonomic teams—much as many workplaces have quality teams and safety teams. In fact, he sees these teams as closely related. Good ergonomics means more safety and better quality, he says.

A useful training program will cover at least the following components:

- Why special equipment is needed
  —What health concerns it addresses
  —What risk factors it is designed to control or eliminate

- When the equipment should be used

- Who should use the equipment

- How to use the equipment

- How to determine whether you are using the equipment properly

• What else might be done to complement the ergonomic benefits of the equipment

• Who is available to answer questions that might come up

If you work in a job that might be high risk and you have not been properly trained, you may be using your chairs, tools, or other equipment improperly. The information in this book can help you find answers for some of your questions, but you may need to ask your supervisor or employer to help.

A second way ergonomic training can be useful is in helping workers become more aware of how they are "using themselves"—what movements or postures they may be making that could contribute to CTDs. Could you hold a tool less tightly? Do you need to flex your hand when you reach for a part that you are installing? Is there a way to set up your work area so that you can reach the computer mouse more easily?

Misuse is too often overlooked in training programs. Considerable attention is paid to ergonomic solutions and job design components such as rest breaks, while individual characteristics are generally considered to be a given and ignored.

Dainoff, a highly respected researcher on computer-related health problems and solutions, uses his own experience with tennis elbow to illustrate this. When he developed tennis elbow (from playing tennis), his doctor's prescription was not medication or a splint or surgery but tennis lessons.

"He was right," Dainoff reports. The problem was not that he was playing tennis, but that he was doing something wrong when he was playing.

Some people are physically tense and may therefore contract their muscles more quickly and for longer periods than people who are physically loose. In addition, people respond differently to stress. A person who grows anxious when pressed to work quickly is more likely to develop CTDs than is someone who stays calm.

Your personal habits can influence how you are affected by on-the-job CTD risk factors in other ways. Carol Teitelman, a political consultant in Doylestown, Pennsylvania, says that for years she habitually rested her elbows on her desk while talking on the phone. After she started to experience tingling and numbness in her hands, symptoms of a nerve entrapment problem, her doctor urged her to break her habit. When she did, the symptoms subsided.

Training aimed at how you "use" yourself might also include exercises. Some specialists believe that encouraging workers to do exercises suggests that CTDs are caused by workers' physical conditions rather than their working conditions. CTDs are a result of overuse and physical abuse, they contend.

The real value of exercises is that they add a measure of prevention. If only by loosening up your hands and arms before you start work, at a minimum, exercises are a good idea.

For many people, exercises are crucial. "After I started doing exercises my tendinitis seemed to just fade away, even though I kept working at the computer the same as before," a graphic designer reports.

Are CTDs Work-Related?

This may seem to be an odd question in a chapter describing on-the-job risk factors for CTDs. It is, however, an important issue that merits discussion.

A small number of researchers and physicians believe that no relationship has been clearly established between work and CTDs, particularly carpal tunnel syndrome.

Repetitive use of the upper extremity, where the movements involved are comfortable and familiar, does not increase the chances that a worker will develop a musculoskeletal disease, including carpal tunnel syndrome, argues Dr. Norton Hadler of the University of North Carolina at Chapel Hill in the Journal of Occupational Medicine. Dr. Peter Nathan of Portland, Oregon, Hand Surgery and Rehabilitation Center has reached similar conclusions.

Debate on this topic is heated. Contrasting Hadler and Nathan, Dr. Steven Sauter of NIOSH's applied psychology and ergonomic branch says resolutely that "I don't think there is any serious debate on whether CTDs are work-related." The data from NIOSH's extensive health hazard evaluations clearly shows an occupational link to CTDs, he states.

The primary reason for the disagreement is that the two sides use different test methods and different definitions. Nathan, for instance, relies on nerve conduction velocity tests that can detect whether a nerve has lost some of its ability to convey a signal. This happens in advanced cases of carpal tunnel syndrome.

The key here is that nerve conduction velocity

tests cannot usually detect carpal tunnel syndrome until it has reached an advanced stage. That is, the symptoms must be pronounced before they qualify as a case of carpal tunnel syndrome.

A high threshold may have greater scientific validity than, say, the case definition of carpal tunnel syndrome put forth by NIOSH (see page 178). Relying solely on high-threshold tests does not make sense if the goal is to prevent CTD cases and to detect new cases in their early stages, however.

CHAPTER 3
Making Jobs Safer

You can reduce your risk of developing a CTD, but you cannot eliminate the risk altogether. Using the information you collect by evaluating your job and your work environment (see Chapter 2), you should be able to identify aspects of your job that pose potential hazards. The suggestions offered in this chapter can help you make changes to make your job safer.

This chapter consists of three sections. The first section offers principles for prevention, the second gives tips for overcoming obstacles to safer work, and the third describes how experts have proposed solving CTD problems in ten high-risk occupations.

Principles for Preventing CTDs

Many of the principles that occupational safety and health professionals use to address CTD hazards in the workplace are simple and reflect common sense. You can use their principles to help yourself.

Some principles, such as getting proper training and reducing stress, may require the support of your employer. It is important that you know what training you should be getting and what can be done to reduce stress and related psychosocial factors associated with CTDs.

What You Can Do Yourself

Take Rest and Recovery Breaks

All workers need periodic rest breaks. When your work involves high repetition rates, high levels of force, or prolonged periods in one position, rest breaks are essential.

Rest breaks—even very short ones—allow your body to begin recovering from the stress of your work. The human body has a great ability to recuperate. For most jobs, proper rest periods will allow your body to heal itself and prevent CTDs. Work done at a faster pace requires a longer recovery time.

A rest break is not necessarily a coffee break. Use your breaks to get away from the task that is the main activity in your job. Often this occurs naturally. A secretary may spend several hours a day working at a computer, but that time is usually broken up by phone calls, visitors, and other duties. At assembly line jobs, however, rest breaks sometimes are strictly scheduled.

There are a few things you should do during your rest break: change your position, take a walk or stretch your legs, do some exercises (see below), and take a few deep breaths. In addition, make it a habit during your rest breaks to take note of any unusual sensations, particularly those that might indicate early signs of CTDs.

The timing and length of your rest breaks depend on your work. A good general guideline is to take at least one fifteen-minute break from your main task every two hours. If you are doing intensive work— such as polishing cars all day with a hand buffer—you should take at least one ten-minute break every hour. Overworked muscles take longer to recover and short "mini-breaks" seem to improve your body's ability to recover.

Exercises

Many CTD specialists believe that you have as much reason to warm up before starting work as professional athletes do. If the physical demands of your job are sufficient to make you concerned about CTDs, you owe it to yourself to develop an on-the-job exercise program.

Exercises prepare you for physical exertion by increasing blood flow to the muscles and by signaling the muscles, tendons, and ligaments that they are going to be used.

A practical exercise regimen will not take a lot of

time. You can do most exercises while you are sitting or standing near your desk. The photos and text on the following pages are suggestions for some simple exercises you can try.

Do these exercises gently. You can stretch your muscles by working with soft, small movements as well as you can with hard, large movements, and you do not have to strain yourself to exercise.

If you have been treated for a CTD, particularly if you have been given exercises by a physical therapist or an occupational therapist, you can use the exercises you learned during treatment.

You will be better off if you do gentle exercises before starting your work and regularly through the day than you will if you only stretch out once in the morning. Use any spare moment to do one or more of the exercises. It is not essential that you do a complete series.

In addition, the benefits of exercise do not eliminate the need for rest breaks, properly designed and installed equipment, healthy work practices, and safe job organizations.

Exercises are not for everyone, however. If you have a nerve-related CTD—carpal tunnel syndrome, thoracic outlet syndrome, ulnar nerve entrapment at the wrist, or ulnar nerve entrapment at the elbow—exercises can do more harm than good. This is also true if you have a CTD that has reached an advanced state. As a general precaution, if you already have a CTD you should consult with a health professional before trying any exercises.

Hand Stretch

Clench your fist firmly and hold it clenched for about three seconds, then open your hand and fan your fingers as widely as you can manage comfortably. Hold this open position for three seconds, as well.

Repeat this cycle five times.

This simple exercise helps to overcome the effects of keeping your hands in a single position for a long time, such as when you type at a computer keyboard or when you hold a tool.

Wrist Extension Stretch

Put the palms of your hands together in front of you at about the level of your chest (see photo). Press your

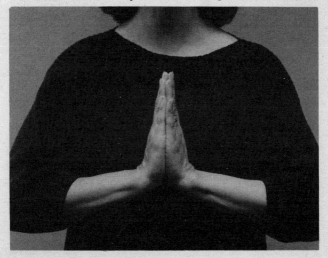

Wrist Extension Stretch

hands together gently and evenly. Hold this position for five seconds, and relax. Repeat five times. This can be done either sitting or standing.

Wrist Flexion Stretch

Put your arm straight in front of you, as if you are pointing directions. Make sure that your elbow is fully extended but not locked. Flex your wrist gently (bend it toward the palm). Use your other hand to pull the flexed hand toward your body (see photo). Pull for five seconds, release your flexed hand, and let your arm rest at your side. Repeat five times.

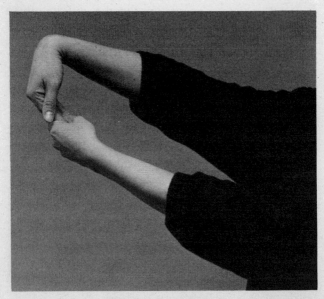

Wrist Flexion Stretch

Wrist Strengthening

Here is a series of four exercises you can do to develop strength in your wrists and the muscles in your arms. All four require you to use one hand to offer resistance to the other.

For each exercise, make a loose fist with your wrist in a neutral position and follow the instructions given here. Do each exercise for about five seconds, and repeat the series five times.

• With your palm facing *up,* cover your fist with your other hand and press down gradually and firmly for five seconds. Resist this pressure with your fist (see photo).

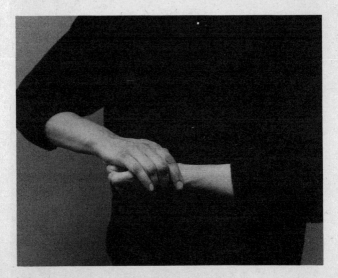

Wrist Strengthening

• With your palm facing *down*, cover your fist and press. Resist (see photo).

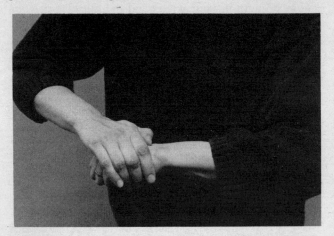

• With your *thumb* facing up, cover your thumb and fist and press down. Resist (see photo).

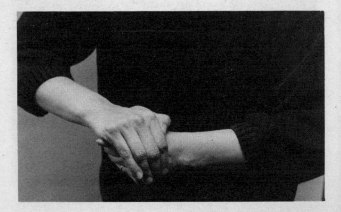

• With your thumb facing *down,* use your free hand to press against the knuckles of your fist. Resist (see photo).

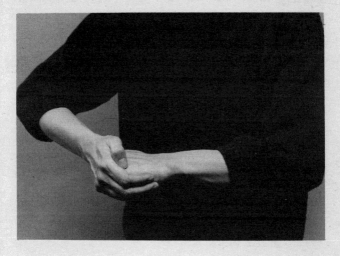

Shoulder Rolls

In a standing position, rotate your shoulder joint in a circle. Do five circles in one direction and five circles in the other direction. Repeat five times.

Arm Circles

In a standing position with your arms held straight out to your sides, rotate your arms at the shoulder joint. Do at least ten small circles and gradually make them larger. Reverse the direction of the circles, working from large circles to small ones. Repeat three times.

Be careful to do this gently—do not swing your arms so hard that you risk damaging the shoulder joint or pulling yourself off balance. In addition, before starting, make sure that you have plenty of room to swing your arms without hitting anything.

Arm Stretch

This exercise should be done while sitting. It stretches muscles and loosens the joints in your back and neck as well as in your arms, wrists, and hands.

Clasp your hands together in front of you and reach your clasped hands toward the sky. Let your hands and arms sway gently to one side. Try not to lean either forward or backward with your body while you do this. When you are leaning as far as you can comfortably, hold that position for three seconds. Sway to the other side and hold that position for three seconds.

Repeat five times.

Back and Shoulder Arch

This stretch primarily benefits your shoulders and neck.

While seated, clasp your hands behind your head and lean back slowly. Let the back of your chair provide support. When you have leaned as far as you can comfortably, hold that position for up to five seconds. Return to an upright position and repeat three times.

Shoulder Pendulum

Stand with your right hand holding on to a chair. Using the chair as a support, let your left arm dangle from the shoulder joint, swaying gently. Try to feel the weight of your arm as gravity pulls on it. Continue this, keeping your arm swaying, as long as it feels comfortable. Switch arms.

Tennis Elbow Stretch

Hold your hand up as if you are waving to someone (see photo on page 70). Slowly roll your fingers into a loose fist, continue rolling your hand so that your wrist flexes. Keeping this position, extend your elbow so that your arm is fully extended in front of you. Hold this position for three seconds, and then let your arm rest at your side for five seconds. Repeat five times.

Use Tools That Fit You and Your Job

One of the fundamental ideas behind ergonomics is that the equipment should fit the person who will use it. In general, this means that handles on pliers, power tools, and other equipment should allow the operator to use them without putting his wrist, elbow, or shoulder in an awkward posture and without putting unnecessary pressure on any part of the body.

Common problems include tools that are made for use by one hand but not the other, those with handles that require awkward grips either because they are too small or too large, and those that are slippery or otherwise hard to hold. Any of these problems could lead to a CTD.

Your tools and equipment should not require extreme force. In jobs that do require force, mechanical

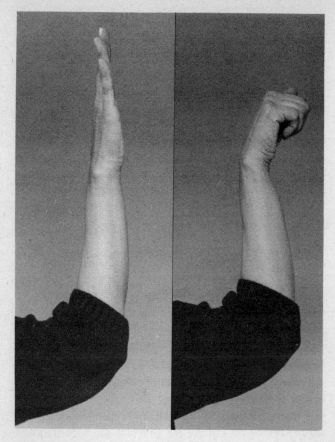

Tennis Elbow Stretch

devices should be used to reduce the work load on the worker. Workers deboning chicken breasts in a poultry processing plant put strain on their arms and hands. A simple solution is a mechanically assisted

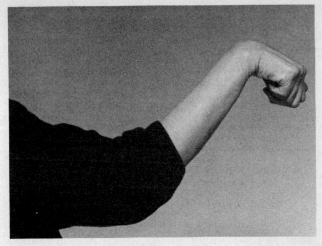

Tennis Elbow Stretch

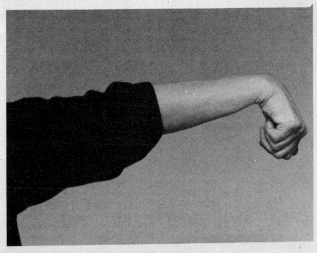

Tennis Elbow Stretch

tool that pulls the chicken meat away from the bone so that the worker can cut it easily.

Use "jigs" and fixtures whenever possible to hold your work in place. (A jig is a guide or stand.) By mounting an object on a jig, you can rotate it or tilt it as needed to eliminate awkward positions.

Any time you can replace a hand-powered tool with a motor-powered tool, do it. Be alert to the ways that vibration contributes to CTDs, however. Just because the motor is doing the work for you does not always mean that it is safer.

Computer keyboards comprise another common type of tool that can be changed to fit the workers and their jobs. According to ergonomist Marvin Dainoff, twenty-two different models of so-called alternative design keyboards are either in development or already on the market. They range from a fairly conventional model to multipart keyboards that use key "chords" to enter data much as court stenographer's devices do.

Apple Computer has introduced a model that is split in the middle and pivots up to thirty degrees along a hinge at the back to allow users to type without bending their wrists toward their small fingers (ulnar deviation). Other alternative keyboards allow the user to adjust them to almost any position and angle.

These keyboards are new and there are no research data proving that they will reduce CTDs. Most manufacturers emphasize this and assert only that the keyboards improve comfort.

Several ergonomists have commented favorably but

cautiously. Dr. Thomas Armstrong of the University of Michigan told *VDT News* (January/February 1993) that the Apple keyboard is a step in the right direction, but emphasized that ulnar deviation is just one of many potential risk factors.

NIOSH is currently conducting a study of several alternative keyboards that may help clarify whether they are beneficial, but the lead researcher, Dr. Naomi Swanson, points out that this research will not prove whether these sorts of devices will prevent injuries.

Know How to Adjust and Use Your Equipment

It is not enough that a tool or piece of equipment is adjustable—it must be *easy* to adjust. Modern office chairs may be the most common example of equipment with all the advantages and all the pitfalls that ergonomics can offer. Some chairs adjust to almost every imaginable position, but you feel as if you need an operator's license to use them.

Marvin Dainoff calls this the "degrees of freedom" problem—if you have the freedom to adjust every major component on your chair any way you like, how do you decide which adjustments are the right ones? You could spend half of your work day making minor adjustments.

More likely, however, you will be overwhelmed by the options and not even try to adjust your chair.

Ask for and learn how to use tools and equipment that are properly adjusted to the task at hand. In the meat cutting industry, a common cause of CTDs is the ulnar deviation (bending your wrist toward your little finger) that accompanies slicing with a knife.

To solve this problem, ergonomists developed a knife with a blade that extends at a right angle from the handle, which straps around the back of the hand. This enables meat cutters to use the knife with minimal gripping force and it puts the blade at an angle that eliminates ulnar deviation. What makes the design particularly effective is that it can use different, interchangeable blades to reduce the strain of different cutting motions. But the meat cutters will not benefit if they have not learned which blade to use when.

Maintenance

An electric power tool that is out of whack will vibrate. A knife that is dull requires extra muscular force to make cuts. A computer keyboard that is dirty may have keys that stick.

Good maintenance of equipment is one of the easiest things to overlook, but it also is one of the easiest things to do. Make sure that you know how to maintain your tools and equipment.

What You and Your Employer Should Do

Training

When you start a new job that involves CTD risk factors, you should receive training in:

- What the risk factors are on your job

- What you can do to reduce your risk

• What the employer will do if your equipment or tools are inappropriate or dangerous

• Who in the management team is responsible for health and safety

• Who is responsible for workers' compensation and disability insurance—the employer or you

Job Design

Changing the organization and structure of jobs can reduce repetition, stress, and other CTD risk factors. Here are some ways to improve your job:

• *Combine jobs to reduce repetitive tasks.* Two or more jobs that involve repetitive tasks can be combined in many instances to add variety to the work.

• *Allow workers to rotate jobs.* A good way to reduce the cumulative effects of repetitive motions is to organize the workplace so that workers can rotate jobs. Some employers prefer to automate highly repetitive tasks to eliminate hazards. Unfortunately, this can also eliminate the job.

• *Give workers as much decision-making latitude as possible.* Workers who feel they have some control over the content of their jobs will experience less stress. They also will feel that their contribution is meaningful.

• *Allow workers to pace themselves.* Using computers to set the work pace or to monitor productivity forces workers into highly routine conditions and eliminates naturally occurring rest breaks. It also causes high levels of stress.

• *Allow frequent rest breaks or pauses.* In jobs where the workers do not control their own schedules, employers and supervisors should build in rest breaks or pauses.

• *Give new employers a chance to adjust.* A new worker who is still learning a job could begin to develop a CTD trying to keep up with a demanding work pace. When she is more comfortable with the tasks the job involves, she will naturally work faster.

Overcoming Obstacles to Safer Work

You need to be realistic about what changes you can expect at your job. Making changes in the workplace can produce resistance from your co-workers, your supervisor, or your employer. There are no simple answers when this happens. If you belong to a labor union or if your company has a health and safety committee or a quality assurance committee, ask these groups for help.

Your co-workers might feel that you are trying to "rock the boat" or that you are not a team player. In many workplaces, particularly blue-collar ones, there is a belief that pain is part of the job.

Other co-workers may fear reprisal for complaining. At three U.S. Postal Service facilities, according to a study done for OSHA, workers with symptoms of CTDs said they never reported them because other workers had been penalized for doing so.

Many employers greet CTD complaints skeptically, though recognition that the problem is real is up from only a few years ago. They suspect that the disorders do not exist or that the worker submitting the complaint is either a malingerer or is angry about something that happened on the job.

A senior editor at the Los Angeles *Times* told the *Columbia Journalism Review* that management's views have changed since the mid-1980s: "[O]ur medical staff back then thought it was a scam. One even called it 'mass hysteria.' But no one thinks that now. The problem is real, and it's in every newspaper's interest to deal with it." More than 400 CTD-related workers' compensation claims have been filed by *Times* employees, and a company spokeswoman says that the cost of these claims is more than $2.2 million. By comparison, the paper spent $1.5 million on new ergonomic computer equipment to improve working conditions.

One of the best ways to introduce your concerns to your employer is to emphasize the fact that your productivity is suffering due to your working conditions and that you have some ideas about how to improve both. Research done at NIOSH in Cincinnati, Ohio shows, for example, that workers who take more breaks—and spend less time actually doing their jobs—are more productive than workers with fewer rest breaks. Several other studies have also found that workers with ergonomically correct equipment are consistently more productive by as much as 25 percent.

The Occupational Safety and Health Act requires employers to provide safe working conditions. In the late 1980s, as federal statistics showed CTDs rising rapidly, OSHA stepped up its enforcement efforts to reduce the number of new CTD cases. The agency issued a series of multimillion-dollar fines that got the attention of many companies.

But OSHA's enforcement staff is short-handed and your chances for safer working conditions are better if you can negotiate safety changes with your employer. Caroline Rose, an editor with tendinitis who has helped organize a loose network of CTD suffers, points out that most employers would rather work things out with you than face a lawsuit.

Ergonomist Marvin Dainoff believes that the key to improving working conditions rests with employers and managers. Management must do four things, he believes:

• Recognize that CTDs are a serious problem.

• Involve employees in decisions.

• Train workers, because if you help people understand the condition they will become your best ally.

• Encourage formation of ergonomic teams to evaluate working conditions and suggest improvements on an ongoing basis.

He warns that the issue that may ultimately make employers take action is medical and insurance costs. "When you start talking about the huge costs of health care, then you have a motivation," he explains.

David Eisen, research director for the Newspaper Guild, a union, agrees. He says that management in general has been "very slow to respond. Management starts to get responsive when it starts to receive large disability claims." The guild represents editors and reporters at some 200 newspapers, magazines, and radio and television stations in the United States and Canada. CTDs have become major health problems at as many as 100 publications and stations, he says, including the Fresno, California, *Bee,* New York *Newsday,* the *New York Times,* and the Los Angeles *Times.*

Eisen feels management is coming around. "We're beginning to see a change," he says.

Real-life Solutions in Ten High-Risk Industries

Hypothetical answers are best saved for hypothetical problems. To help you put your knowledge to work in the real world, the final section of this chapter tells you how some of the nation's top CTD safety specialists have tried to solve CTD problems in ten different occupations using the principles just described.

All of the cases are drawn from work done by the federal government. As you read these recommendations, keep in mind the fact that not all of them were carried out. Real solutions sometimes meet real resistance and real obstacles.

Prevention: Computer Use

The high rate of CTDs among employees of US West Communications has received more attention than perhaps any other cluster.

In July 1989, the company and the Communications Workers of America together asked NIOSH to investigate reports of high CTD rates. NIOSH officials undertook one of the most thorough workplace evaluations of CTDs yet done.

A total of 518 US West employees working in offices in Phoenix, Minneapolis, and Denver participated in the study. Of these, 111 (22 percent) had one or more CTDs diagnosed by physical examinations—15 percent had tendon-related illnesses (tendinitis, tenosynovitis), 4 percent had carpal tunnel syndrome or other nerve entrapment illnesses, 8 percent had muscle-related ailments, 3 percent had joint-related disorders, and another 3 percent had ganglion cysts.

While the original concern focused on directory assistance telephone operators, NIOSH included other groups of workers using computers in the study population. This enabled the researchers to make comparisons among groups and thus to evaluate a larger number of potential contributing factors.

Perhaps the most significant element of the NIOSH investigation was that the investigators found high CTD rates despite the fact that the physical working conditions at US West were considered good. Most of the workstations evaluated were "ergonomically correct," NIOSH noted.

This led the research team to focus on the possible role psychosocial factors may play in CTD cases. For this reason, the study breaks new ground and its recommendations are unique in the field:

Recommendations

• In changing psychosocial factors on the job, the study recommended taking into account:

—*Job security*. Reduce ambiguity about career development and opportunities. Inform workers about promotion possibilities and impending organizational changes.

—*Work pressure*. Look for causes of pressure. The available research literature can be used to identify possible causes and prevention strategies.

—*Job diversity*. Give employees work that involves a range of tasks or activities, as well as the chance to make decisions and exercise latitude in their jobs. Do not overload workers with too much diversity or too many decisions.

—*Support*. Encourage supervisory and co-worker support.

—*Information processing*. Be aware that some jobs, particularly computer-based ones, can require workers to manage overwhelming amounts of data. Reduce these loads, as they are called, where possible.

—*Work surges*. Organize and manage work so that individual workers are not swamped by unexpected surges in their jobs.

• Reduce the number of keystrokes, where possible. In some jobs, this can be done by adapting the way the work is organized. For example, instead of requiring workers to enter strings of numbers more than once, computer software could simplify this procedure so that the numbers are entered only once and subsequently verified by a single keystroke.

• Use work organization changes to reduce stress. These might include rest breaks away from the computer, job designs that require workers to stand periodically, replacing computer-paced systems with self-paced work, and job rotation.

• Replace work station equipment that is ergonomically improper with new, correct equipment.

• Promptly evaluate all reported cases of possible CTDs. Employees should receive medical care without a threat of fear or reprisal by the employer.

• Use joint employer-union (or employee) ergonomics committees to identify new or existing hazards, to suggest solutions, and evaluate the effectiveness of attempted solutions.

Source: Health Hazard Evaluation Report (HETA 89-299-2230), "US West Communications, Phoenix, AZ, Minneapolis, MN, Denver, CO," July 1992, National Institute for Occupational Safety and Health, Cincinnati, Ohio.

Prevention: Meat Cutting

Few, if any, occupations are more closely linked to CTDs than meat cutting. The American Federation of Labor–Congress of Industrial Organizations (AFL-CIO) has estimated that one of every seven meat cutters will develop a CTD. This includes not only workers in slaughterhouses and packinghouses but butchers at grocery stores and delicatessens, as well.

Many meat cutting jobs require high levels of force to cut meat (particularly when knives are not well maintained), awkward positions needed to gain leverage for cutting, high repetition rates as workers make the same series of cuts over and over, and cold temperatures that can affect joints, tendons, and muscles.

Some employers have failed to make workplace changes to reduce CTDs. In 1988, OSHA fined two major meat packers, John Morrell & Company of Sioux City, South Dakota, and IBP, Inc., of Dakota City, Nebraska, $4.3 million and $5.7 million, respectively, for working conditions that contributed to CTDs. Rather than pay the whole fine, IBP reached an agreement with the United Food and Commercial Workers (UFCW) and OSHA that significantly reduced the penalty but required the company to make major changes in its equipment and work practices. Such negotiated reductions of OSHA penalties are common.

OSHA has recognized that the CTD problem is common across the industry. In 1990, the Labor Department said that CTDs and related illnesses were ten times as common in meat cutting as in the general public. That year, under considerable pressure from labor unions to issue a binding regulation, OSHA instead released a set of guidelines for reducing CTDs in this industry. Union officials contend that the guidelines are inadequate because they leave too much discretion to employers. Nonetheless, the guidelines comprise the most extensive and most aggressive stand to combat work-related CTDs taken so far by a public agency. The major points of these recommendations are summarized as follows.

Recommendations

• Management should make a high-level commitment to a program that can significantly reduce CTDs. Top company officials should give health and safety the same level of importance as production.

• The program should be written and it should be clearly communicated to workers. It should set clear goals and include objectives toward meeting those goals.

• Employees should be involved in the CTD safety program. One of the things included in the IBP-UFCW agreement mentioned earlier is deputization of a group of employees as ergonomics monitors to detect hazards.

• A CTD management program should include four elements:

—*Work site analysis.* This might include use of an ergonomic checklist, review of company medical records, screening surveys of workers, and recommendations for preventing CTDs.

—*Hazard prevention and control.* This should include ergonomic and related equipment design changes, improved work practices involving such things as a "conditioning" period for new employees, protection against hazards (for example, proper gloves to reduce exposure to cold temperatures without compromising grip strength), and job design and performance modifications ranging from reducing the number of repetitive motions to programs for maintaining sharp knives.

—*Medical management.* Trained medical professionals should take active roles in preventing CTDs, including making workplace tours to identify potential hazards. Early detection should be emphasized. OSHA also suggested a detailed protocol for medical evaluation and treatment.

—*Training and education.* Both general training about CTDs and their risk factors, as well as job-specific training about ways to limit CTD hazards, are recommended. Managers and supervisors also should receive training.

Source: "Ergonomics Program Management Guidelines for Meatpacking Plants" (OSHA 3123), 1990, Occupational Safety and Health Administration, U.S. Department of Labor.

Is Your CTD Safety Program "The Real Thing"?

As concern about CTDs continues to grow, some workers and labor unions caution that companies are offering CTD safety programs that are ineffective and that divert employees from getting proper medical care.

In 1989, the United Food and Commercial Workers (UFCW) union's national health and safety office issued an internal report warning about "gimmick-type approaches that may sound good, but do little to prevent" CTDs.

The UFCW cautioned against efforts to change workers rather than working conditions, job rotation programs that are not based on the advice of trained specialists, and hot wax hand and wrist treatments that temporarily reduce pain but can worsen CTDs by increasing swelling.

The UFCW also outlined the components of an effective CTD safety program. Workers should be involved in ergonomic and other CTD-related decisions, specialists hired by meat cutting companies to redesign working conditions should have proper training, and all workers should be trained to identify CTD risk factors and prevention methods. New workers should have specially designed training and gradual "conditioning" periods.

In addition, the union urged an "aggressive" medical program that seeks to detect CTD cases early. Medical care should be provided without delay, follow-up should be aggressive and regular, and medical professionals should have the authority to reassign affected workers to jobs that pose less risk of causing CTDs.

Prevention: Postal Work

The U.S. Postal Service is the largest nondefense employer in the nation, and its use of automated equipment to improve mail processing has put it at the center of the CTD problem.

The primary problems in the postal service are letter sorting machines (LSMs), which have keyboards that workers use to separate incoming batches of mail for sorting and delivery. Various types of keyboards have been used since LSMs were first installed in the 1960s, but all generally require operators to type in a series of numbers at a rate of about one series per second. A conveyor system brings a single piece of mail in front of the operator, who must read the address and zip code and enter the appropriate code into the sorting machine. Adding to the pressure of the job is the fact that many of the letters the LSM operators must sort have been rejected by the postal service's automated optical character recognition system, most often because the addresses are not clearly written.

The American Postal Workers Union has estimated that the average LSM operator makes fifteen million or more keystrokes a year, or on the order of sixty thousand keystrokes per working day. The postal service employs about fifty thousand LSM operators.

An accurate CTD rate among LSM operators is hard to come by, in part because the postal service is not required to report data to OSHA as private employers must do. Many health surveys of LSM operators have been done, however, and the CTD rates are consistently high. A 1981 NIOSH evaluation found that 54 percent of LSM operators had developed CTDs. Other studies have found CTD rates between 18 and 40 percent.

The postal service has a history of not responding to CTD findings and the concerns of its workers, and as recently as a 1991 congressional hearing contended that it was "premature" to begin a program for controlling CTDs. In addition, at three postal service centers supervisors have reportedly punished workers for reporting CTD symptoms, effectively creating a climate of fear that discouraged other workers from reporting symptoms.

The following recommendations are compiled from several of the studies that have been done concerning postal employees and CTDs.

Recommendations

• Operators should spend fifteen minutes doing non-LSM tasks for every thirty minutes they spend working on the sorting machine. This time structure produced fewer sorting errors and significantly higher productivity than did a forty-five-minute/fifteen-minute structure in one study.

• Reduce the pacing of the LSM system so that operators' keying rates would be decreased. Consider making LSM jobs self-paced instead of machine-paced.

• Make jobs more diverse so that LSM operators spend less time at these machines and more time doing other tasks.

• Add an error key that allows operators to reenter numbers when they make a mistake. This could significantly reduce the performance pressure.

• Provide equipment that is properly designed for ergonomic purposes. Keyboards should be fully adjustable; wristrests, armrests, and footrests should be provided; and chairs should offer better support in the seat and back.

• Reduce or eliminate overtime, if possible.

• Improve training of workers to make them more aware of CTD risk factors, symptoms, and prevention methods.

• Step up medical surveillance to increase detection of CTDs at early stages.

Prevention: Supermarket Checkers

In July 1989, investigators from NIOSH began to study reports that supermarket checkers at a chain of grocery stores in New Jersey and New York were experiencing higher than normal rates of CTDs. The reports were made by the local affiliate of the United Food and Commercial Workers union (UFCW).

From 28 stores in the Shoprite chain, the NIOSH team selected four—Fooderama's Shoprite in Bricktown, New Jersey, Big V's Shoprite in Middletown, New York, Wakefern's Shoprite in Clark, New Jersey, and Fooderama's Shoprite in Sayreville, New Jersey. All but the Sayreville store used laser scanners at the checkouts, and all had scales set up higher than the conveyer belt and scanner.

The employees at the four stores were asked to undergo physical examinations and to answer questionnaires about their physical condition, work history, hobbies, and medical history. There were 319 employees who participated, from which 281 were used for analysis.

"CTDs of the hand and wrist were the most common problem found on examination for both checkers and noncheckers," NIOSH concluded in its report on the study. In addition, looking more closely, NIOSH found that "there was a statistically significant association between checking and having a CTD."

More important, the investigators determined that the length of employment was statistically significantly associated with hand CTDs, neck CTDs, and carpal tunnel syndrome. Finally, the study found that using laser scanners was linked to CTDs.

Recommendations

NIOSH's main recommendations are:

• Place the keyboard in front of the cashier and above the scanner. The keyboard should be tiltable in all directions and should be no higher than the checker's shoulder.

• Locate the scale and the scanner in front of the cashier. This could be done by locating the scanner inside the scale or by using a vertical scanner.

• The scale should be flush with the conveyor belt to eliminate twisting and reaching to weigh produce.

• Scanners should be capable of reading universal product code labels from most surfaces. Many scanners require the checker to twist and turn products to get the scanner to read them properly.

• For a conveyer height of thirty-four to thirty-six inches, the outer edge of the scale and the conveyor belt should be within seventeen inches, unless the checker has to reach more than twelve inches. In that case, the conveyor and scale should be within fourteen inches.

• Put a bag stand beside the checker with the top of the bag even with the conveyor belt so that the checker can immediately bag items after scanning them. This would reduce approximately by half the number of times the checker must lift and maneuver items.

• Have a second person do the bagging, where possible. This will significantly reduce the number of repetitious movements and awkward postures for the checker. It also will provide "micro" rest breaks.

• Provide an adjustable sit/stand bar or seat in the checkstand area. This will enable the checker to rest during lulls in the work cycle, such as when a customer is writing a check.

• Checkers should learn to eliminate unnecessary motions, such as:
  —Reaching across the conveyer to unload or load items from customers' carts
  —Tying full plastic grocery bags before giving them to customers
  —Reaching for items and pulling the across the scanner instead of waiting for the conveyor belt to bring the times to the edge of the scanner.
  —Scanning an item multiples times rather than keying in multiple purchases of a single item (for example, scanning six bottles of soda separately rather than having the scanner count one scan six times)

Source: Health Hazard Evaluation Report (HETA 88-344-2092), "Shoprite Supermarkets, New Jersey–New York," January 1991, National Institute for Occupational Safety and Health, Cincinnati, Ohio.

Prevention: Newspaper Employees

Employees at the Melville, New York, and New York City offices of *Newsday,* a daily newspaper serving Long Island and New York City, were reporting what appeared to be high rates of CTDs in the late 1980s. In May 1989 the publisher and a union representing some of the workers jointly asked NIOSH to evaluate.

The NIOSH researchers relied solely on questionnaire data; no physical examinations were done. They found that 40 percent of the 834 employees who responded to the questionnaire reported symptoms of hand and arm CTDs.

The three factors most clearly associated with CTD incidence, particularly with CTDs of the hand, wrist, forearm, and elbow, were the percentage of work time spent typing, typing speed, and working as a reporter.

"As percent of time typing or typing speed increased, the likelihood of symptoms increased," NIOSH concluded. The investigation team could not determine what it was about typing speed that linked it to CTDs, but they hypothesized that it "may be related to the effort to type faster and increased muscle tension."

The NIOSH team also was unable to determine why being a reporter put a person at risk. "It is possible that perceived work pressure may be a factor," they suggested. "A proposed mechanism is that work pressure may lead to increased muscle tension which may, in turn, lead to increased muscle fatigue and symptoms."

Recommendations

• Consider work organization changes such as rest breaks for reporters and editors away from their computer jobs. Reorganize jobs so that employees do not have to work at their computers for long, uninterrupted periods.

• Provide proper, adjustable chairs, wrist and other supports, and equipment for all employees.

• Train employees on the proper use of the adjustable equipment. Evaluate how the equipment is being used.

• Provide proper medical management for workers with CTDs.

• Set up a joint labor-management ergonomics committee. The committee would make decisions about purchasing new equipment and about the success or failure of attempted solutions.

• Train the ergonomics committee in health and ergonomic hazard surveillance and workplace and job evaluation techniques.

• Consider retesting employees for CTD symptoms after one year.

Source: Health Hazard Evaluation Report (HETA 89-250-2046), "Newsday, Inc., Melville, NY," June 1990, National Institute for Occupational Safety and Health, Cincinnati, OH.

Prevention: Fish Processing

The Point Adams Packing Company (PAPCO) of Hammond, Oregon, is a commercial fish packing plant that employed 145 production workers in June 1983, when NIOSH investigators visited the facility.

The company had found in its lost-work-time accident records for 1981 and 1982 what appeared to be an excessive number of cases of carpal tunnel syndrome, tendinitis, and other CTDs. For those two years, CTDs made up 20 percent of the company's reportable accidents under OSHA's reporting system and 80 percent of the lost workdays.

The CTD cases were concentrated in three job categories: filleters, trimmers, and slimers (the term used to describe workers who butcher black cod).

The filleters' job was to hold a fish with a pinch grip (using primarily the fingers) while first slicing it open and then removing the fillet. "The cutting process requires a variety of hand positions, with mild to moderate ulnar deviation [bending toward the little finger], accompanied by more or less continual flexion [bending toward the palm] of the knife hand," NIOSH explained.

NIOSH noted that the cutting motions for filleting were "complex" and involved numerous high-risk positions. Since the fish were kept on ice before they came to the filleters, they were partially frozen and cutting required high force. In addition, the work environment was kept cool to prolong the freshness of the fish. Gloves made partially of wire mesh to protect against cuts were often worn on the hand that held the fish, making it an awkward process that required considerable grip force.

Many of the filleters worked with elevated shoulders and elbows held away from their sides. "This appeared to be a very stressful position to maintain," the researchers reported. The NIOSH team also found the filleters fully extending their arms periodically to grab or dispose trays of fish.

The filleters were rated on the basis of their productivity and the rating was used to recall the best filleters for more work. "This recall system placed emphasis on high productivity whereby workers tended to ignore or tolerate repetitive motion-type injuries," according to the researchers. In addition, there were no formal work hours—the filleters and everyone else worked until the day's haul was processed.

Trimmers removed scales, gills, or other unwanted parts from the filleted fish. NIOSH concluded that this job is not as physically demanded as filleting.

Slimers, who were selected on the basis of seniority rather than productivity, could be assigned to any of three jobs that were part of the process. Because of the seniority system and because sliming was not done every day, it was considered by NIOSH to involve "relatively less mental and physical stress" than filleting.

When the NIOSH team observed the workers on the job, they concluded that a primary problem appeared to be the design of the knife handles being used. Through an arrangment with an outside researcher, they developed specifications for an optimal knife handle, but they could not locate a knife that fit their criteria.

Not surprisingly, the investigators concluded that high work rates, awkward hand and wrist positions and motions, gloves that compromise grip strength, cold temperature, use of high forces for prolonged periods, excessive reaching, improper work surface heights, and improper tool handle design contributed to the CTD problem at PAPCO.

Recommendations

• The optimum handle size is 5 inches in length by 2 inches in width by 0.8 inches in thickness. This is about twice the size of the handles in use at PAPCO.

• The cutting table should be thirty-two to thirty-eight inches above the workers' feet, depending on the height of the workers.

• The work area should be reorganized so that employees do not have to reach with fully extended arms holding trays of fish.

• The cutting table surface should be textured to increase friction and reduce the force needed to hold the fish steady for cutting.

• Gloves should fit properly. Despite the fact that the gloves make it more difficult to grip the fish firmly, they should continue to be used because of the coldness of the fish and the working environment.

• New employees should be trained to minimize the types of movements and postures that are associated with CTDs.

• New employees should apprentice with experienced filleters to learn (1) proper knife angles for minimizing force requirements and (2) how to properly sharpen a knife.

• Slimers should use a mechanical guillotine-type device to decapitate black cod. This task was found to require considerable force.

Source: Health Hazard Evaluation Report (HETA 83-251-1685), "Point Adams Packing Company, Hammond, OR," April 1986, National Institute for Occupational Safety and Health, Cincinnati, Ohio.

Prevention: Grinding and Cutting

In 1981, while General Motors was reconfiguring its plant in Framingham, Massachusetts, to prepare for production of a new car line, nineteen out of one hundred workers involved in tearing out an old conveyor system and installing a new one reported CTD-like symptoms. The symptoms included numbness and tingling in the hands, suggesting a nerve-related disorder.

All of the workers used power grinding and cutting tools regularly, usually for ten-hour shifts, six days a week. Both the cutting and grinding involved awkward postures—either stooping, squatting, or kneeling when the work was being done at ground level, or reaching overhead when the work was being done at the ceiling of the plant and the workers were standing on lifts.

Constructing the new conveyor involved welding, so the NIOSH team sent in to investigate was concerned about the possibility that airborne chemicals may have been causing neurological damage. Air quality tests discounted this hypothesis.

The investigators concluded that the workers' symptoms were caused by nerve injuries. "Specific work postures which appeared to be significant in terms of the development of the traumatic injuries include wrist flexion and extension, and radial and ulnar deviations to weld, grind, and cut metal. These positions resulted in repetitive trauma to upper extremities," they reported.

In addition, they suspected that prolonged periods of holding heavy tools at or above chest level may have led to thoracic outlet syndrome, the compression of the nerves and blood vessels as they exit from the upper chest into the arm. "Furthermore, repetitive local vibration stress occurred." They concluded that none of the cases involved permanent damage.

Recommendations

• Use tools with reduced vibrations.

• Wear gloves made of materials that absorb vibration and reduce its impact on the hand.

• Use grinding tools that allow the wrist to stay in a neutral position.

• Hold tools with only as much force (tightness) as needed. Unnecessarily tight grips increase the amount of vibration transferred from the tools to the hands and arms.

• When power tools must be lifted overhead, workers should lower their arms frequently for short rests.

Source: Health Hazard Evaluation Report (HETA 81-433-1452), "General Motors Corporation, Framingham, MA," May 1984, National Institute for Occupational Safety and Health, Cincinnati, Ohio.

Prevention: Air Filter Manufacturing

Corporate officials at the Donaldson Company, Inc., of Dixon, Illinois, had already identified and proposed preventive measures for a carpal tunnel syndrome problem when NIOSH sent in a team in late 1981 and early 1982.

Between 1975 and 1980, eighteen cases of physician-diagnosed carpal tunnel syndrome were recorded in the company's medical logs. NIOSH was able to contact fifteen of the eighteen and learned that seven CTDs had occurred among workers in just one department at the Donaldson Company. The company had eight departments in all. NIOSH was primarily interested in determining whether any new cases had developed.

The Donaldson Company manufactures air filters

and related parts. In reviewing the production lines, NIOSH identified numerous factors that may have contributed to carpal tunnel syndrome or other CTDs.

The NIOSH researchers also found sixteen possible new cases of carpal tunnel syndrome. These were people who had reported numbness, tingling, or pain in one or both hands since going to work at the Dixon facility. Using questionnaire data obtained from the thirteen possible cases they succeeded in reaching, NIOSH concluded that four had early cases of carpal tunnel syndrome.

Combining the previous fifteen cases and the four new ones, NIOSH observed that all nineteen carpal tunnel syndrome cases occurred among women. Half of the noncases (the balance of the work crew) were men.

After comparing the work histories of the people with carpal tunnel syndrome, the NIOSH team concluded that "new cases appeared to be occurring, with less frequency than in the past, and with a fairly clear relationship to certain work areas." Their final recommendations focused on those areas.

Recommendations

• In a department that involved a repetitive, high-frequency task, repeated ulnar deviation of the wrist, and strain from the physical weight and momentum of a vacuum tool:

—Install an automated system to eliminate the need for the vacuum tool.

—Bend the handle of the vacuum tool to reduce
ulnar deviation of the wrist.
—Reduce the length of the vacuum tool.

• In a department that involved use of an awkward
position over a prolonged period to spray an aerosol
as well as use of needle-nose pliers producing pronounced ulnar deviation:
—Automate the aerosol-spraying routine.
—Substitute bent-handled needle-nose pliers.

• In a department that required force with bent
wrists while cleaning a surface with a putty knife, replace the putty knife with one that has a larger handle.

• In a department that involved (1) continuous gripping with an awkward wrist posture against a handle
trigger to apply a substance (plastisol) using a "pneu-
matic-type" gun, and (2) mechanical rubbing requiring relatively high hand force to remove excess
plastisol:
—Replace the "gun" with one whose trigger did
not require awkward wrist postures.
—Apply the plastisol more carefully to reduce
the amount that must be rubbed off.
—Introduce job rotation, allowing workers to
vary their tasks.

*Source: Health Hazard Evaluation Report (HETA 81-409-1290),
"The Donaldson Company, Inc., Dixon, IL," April 1983, National
Institute for Occupational Safety and Health, Cincinnati, Ohio.*

Prevention: Sewing Uniforms

What do you do when an ergonomic and medical survey finds no *statistical* evidence of job-related CTDs but the rate of reported symptoms among workers is high and the jobs appear to involve high-risk activities? That was the challenge facing a NIOSH team investigating CTDs in 1983 at the United Uniform Company of Memphis, Tennessee.

United Uniform manufactured work uniforms. Of the 125 workers at the plant, 85 to 90 operated sewing machines, making parts of shirts and pants and assembling the parts.

The workers picked up unfinished fabric pieces, aligned them on the sewing machine, and stitched them together. The assembled pieces were put in bins that were within reach so that the workers did not have to get up out of their chairs. According to the NIOSH team, the most common CTD-risk-related activity was ulnar deviation of the wrists among workers using "sleeve-type" sewing machines. Other common activities were pinch grips to lift assembled pieces into bins and abduction of the shoulders to stack finished pieces into piles in the bins.

All of the workers had metal chairs that could not be adjusted and did not not have footrests. Workers who needed higher seats had to use pillows, which in some cases effectively turned the chairs into backless stools.

The NIOSH team separated the workers into low, medium, and high risk categories for two different factors—force and repetition. The researchers rated the level of force by observation and defined the repetition categories as those involving less than seventy-five hundred movements per shift (low risk), seventy-five hundred to twenty thousand movements per shift (medium risk), and more than twenty thousand movements per shift (high risk). Of the forty-seven jobs evaluated, thirteen were low risk, thirty-one were medium risk, and three were high risk.

The researchers observed no statistically significant differences among the job categories in the reported rates of CTD symptoms and concluded that there was no CTD health hazard at United Uniform. Indeed, for some health problems such as hand and wrist numbness, the rate of reported symptoms was higher for the low-risk workers than for the high-risk workers.

How could this be? The answer seems to lie in the fact that most, if not all, of the jobs at United Uniform may have been high-risk in comparison to other types of jobs in other workplaces. The overall rates of symptoms are remarkably high—for instance, for hand and wrist numbness 45 percent of the medium- and high-risk workers reported this symptom and 60 percent of the low-risk group did. For the various CTD symptoms, the rates for low-risk workers ranged from 20 percent to 80 percent.

The NIOSH team seems to have recognized that their data appeared skewed. They reported their findings with an acknowledgment that their lack of a statistical finding was being presented "despite the seemingly frequent occurrence among sewers of symptoms" indicating CTDs.

In addition, the researchers provided an unusually long list of recommendations for a work site at which they had found no problem. They include:

Recommendations

• Sewers using sleeve-type machines should have adjustable chairs with footrests, proper back support, and elbow rests. This will enable them to keep their wrists in a neutral position.

• Make sure that bins used to collect assembled pieces, particularly finished pieces that are heavy, are either emptied regularly or situated so that workers do not have to lift their arms above shoulder height.

• Sewing machine operators who stand should have a footrest and a pad to stand on.

• Bins for unassembled pieces should be designed to reduce the need for pinch grips by allowing workers to slid the pieces out of the bins.

• Use a nonstick material to reduce the friction on some sewing surfaces where large amounts of material must be slid through a sewing machine.

• For sewing that involves joining parts, tilt the work surface slightly away from the workers. This will reduce ulnar deviation and wrist flexion.

• On table-type work surfaces, pad the edges to reduce the potential for pressure on forearms and elbows.

Source: Health Hazard Evaluation Report (HETA 83-205-1702), "United Uniform Company of Memphis," June 1986, National Institute for Occupational Safety and Health, Cincinnati, Ohio.

Prevention: Book Binding

A thorough 1984 NIOSH investigation at the Western Publishing Company of Racine, WI, turned up just 11 cases of carpal tunnel syndrome among a group of 519 workers, or just 2 percent. The cases were confirmed by a physical examination.

At first glance, this hardly seemed to represent a CTD problem, yet the NIOSH team concluded that work-related carpal tunnel syndrome was occurring at seven times the national rate for the printing and publishing industry.

Company records suggested that the carpal tunnel syndrome cases were heavily concentrated in one department at Western—the bindery department, where workers experienced three times as many carpal tunnel syndrome cases as nonbindery employees.

The NIOSH researchers evaluated the ergonomic "stress" of different jobs to try to determine a cause. While the levels were slightly higher for people with carpal tunnel syndrome, this failed to explain the problem. They did identify three factors that seemed to be primary concerns, however: excessive handling of paper in the binding process, poor postures due to inappropriate work station designs, and high levels of force as a result of the weight of the paper.

Work in the bindery involved two types of activities that NIOSH spotlighted. First, binding required workers to handle, fan, jog, and shift large amounts of paper (known as signatures) to maintain quality control. This involved numerous strenuous uses of the arms and hands. Second, workers had to bend and lift the heavy signatures, adding to the wear and tear on the arms and hands.

In other jobs at Western Publishing, the NIOSH researchers observed conditions in need of correction. They addressed these problems, along with those in the bindery department, in their recommendations:

Recommendations

• Teach workers to reduce the amount of paper handling they do. Overhandling of paper and other materials was common.

• Lower stacks of papers or move them to more easily reachable positions so that the workers do not have to reach overhead to grasp heavy loads of paper.

• Lower to below-shoulder height the conveyor belt in the bindery department that carries hardcover books.

• Teach workers who must fan stacks of paper to do so with the bulk of the paper's weight resting on worktables rather than against their bodies.

• Work surfaces for fanning and jogging paper

should be about thirty inches above the floor. Foot stools should be available for short workers or where the work surface is higher than thirty inches.

• In general, provide workers better instruction in proper work practices.

• Encourage job rotation. This might involve changes in job classifications.

• Expand cramped work spaces. Some employees had to lift objects off of conveyor belts in awkward positions.

• Operate an ongoing surveillance program to identify workers with early signs of carpal tunnel syndrome and other CTDs. This effort should not be a substitute for ergonomic and work designs changes.

Source: Health Hazard Evaluation Report (HETA 84-240-1902), "Western Publishing Co., Racine, Wisconsin," June 1988, National Institute for Occupational Safety and Health, Cincinnati, Ohio.

CHAPTER 4

Getting Treatment

Getting proper treatment for your CTD can be a challenge. There is a wide range of opinion among doctors about how and when to diagnose many of the ailments, even the most common ones.

Since physical examinations and other clinical tests cannot reliably detect CTDs until they have advanced to at least a moderately severe state, physicians tend to rely primarily on the self-reported symptoms of patients. This method is often useful, but it can be imprecise. At worst, it can lead to misdiagnoses and improper or inadequate treatments.

When it comes to determining what is causing a CTD, your doctor will have to rely entirely on your observations about your job, your working environment, and your hobbies. Even more than with most medical conditions, your information is critical to an accurate diagnosis.

The rapid rise in the number of reported CTD cases over the past decade caught many physicians by surprise, and not all doctors are fully prepared to recognize and treat these disorders. Dr. Bruce Dickerson of the Occupational Medicine Department at Columbia University in New York City warns that while millions of American workers are at risk, "the medical community is having difficulty diagnosing or even finding these conditions."

The doctors' task is complicated by the lack of a consensus in the research. It is hard to diagnose accurately as long as there is substantial disagreement about how to define a CTD. Even the broad definition for carpal tunnel syndrome proposed by NIOSH (see page 178)—the most useful definition available for any of the job-related CTDs—is not consistently used, for two reasons.

First, most doctors do not know about the NIOSH definition. Second, doctors differ on what tests or information to use to diagnose a carpal tunnel syndrome case, NIOSH's definition notwithstanding. Your physician may rely on self-reported symptoms and working conditions, physical exam results, electrodiagnostic test results such as nerve conduction velocity data, or a combination.

How your doctor evaluates these data could affect your treatment. Judy, who asked that her last name not be used, says she had successful surgery to relieve pressure in the carpal tunnels on both of her wrists in

early 1992 even though the results of her nerve velocity tests "weren't high enough to require surgery." Her
doctor chose to do the operations because of Judy's
reported symptoms. "I couldn't even hold a piece of
paper in my hands," she explains. Judy also told of a
friend who is "in agonizing pain" but whose doctor
refuses to prescribe surgery "because her [nerve conduction velocity] numbers are too low."

Differing treatment approaches are not unusual. For
every patient who feels her doctor waited too long to
do surgery, there is another patient who believes her
doctor should have waited longer.

Effective treatment of other CTDs is compromised
by these diagnostic difficulties. A computer graphics
designer whose doctor had diagnosed tendinitis in the
wrist did not recover until he switched from a mouse
to a track ball to operate his computer. The problem
was not tendinitis, it turned out, but compression of
the ulnar nerve at the wrist, where the man had
pressed on his wrist while using the mouse. Appar-
ently the doctor had not made the distinction because
tendinitis is far more common.

In cases like this, doctors can be limited by the fact
that they do not have access to their patients' workplaces. Job site changes that might prevent a worker
from developing a CTD or reverse his ailment at an
early stage traditionally fall outside of the doctor's authority. The doctor can *recommend* that a patient be
relieved of repetitive tasks, but only the patient and
his employer can resolve that issue.

Some physicians believe doctors should take a

more active role in CTD cases, however. Dr. David Rempel of the University of California at San Francisco, and one of the leading researchers and clinicians on CTDs, published a "special communication" paper in the *Journal of the American Medical Association (JAMA)* to bring physicians and other health professionals up to speed. In it, he urges his colleagues to take an unusually active role in treating CTDs, including "direct involvement in changing the patient's work environment." The physician who follows Rempel's urgings is the rare exception, and the trend in medical insurance toward managed care may further reduce the number of doctors able to take such an active role. In the broader scope of a doctor's daily practice, CTDs are a relatively minor—if increasingly common—ailment. Most doctors simply are not going to give the attention to CTDs that Rempel suggests.

That is why you need to prepare carefully for your visits to your doctor. The initial diagnosis will affect how your condition is treated, whether you will qualify for disability insurance and workers' compensation, and what kind of changes you should make in your job.

By preparing yourself with information and by being assertive about what you believe should be done—using information about your situation from Chapters 2 and 7—you can get the best possible care. As your work with your physician, remember several important things:

• Your doctor will be guided in her examination and diagnosis by the symptoms you report.

• Your doctor does not know anything about your working conditions. Simply reporting that you use a computer a lot is not enough. You must explain your particular working conditions, such as that you sit more or less in one position eight hours and press as many as thirteen thousand keys every hour.

• Be prepared to advocate for a particular type of treatment if you feel it is what you need. For instance, some doctors will try everything before performing carpal tunnel release surgery. Others favor surgery because it is a fairly simple operation that is usually successful.

• Each doctor has a different view of CTDs. If your doctor recommends a different course of treatment than you have in mind, try to understand the reasons. But the decision is yours.

This chapter will help you understand the medical diagnosis and treatment processes for CTDs. It will explain what you should do to prepare for your initial doctor's visit, what your doctor will do to make a diagnosis and why, and what you can expect for treatment.

Before You See Your Doctor

Take as much time as you need to think through your symptoms and your working conditions, and make notes. You may want to use these notes for your own reference when you see your doctor, or you may decide to give your doctor a copy for your medical files.

In addition, these notes may prove useful later if you file a workers' compensation claim. Often in workers' compensation cases, the patient is examined by several doctors, and it can become difficult to remember what your symptoms were when the process started.

The first thing your doctor should do is review your medical history and, as needed, your work history. Here are some questions that can help you prepare for that discussion. They do not cover every possibility, but they will help you to organize your notes:

YOUR SYMPTOMS

When did you first feel something?

Where did/do you feel it?
(It could be more than one place)
   One hand/arm or both
   Fingers
      All
      Little finger and ring finger

Thumb, pointing finger, middle finger and ring
   finger
Base of thumb
Wrist
Forearm
   Near your hand
   Near your elbow
Elbow
   Near the sharp point you make when you bend
      your arm
         On one of the knobs
         On the inside knob
         On the outside knob
Your upper arm
Your shoulder
   The front
   The back
Your entire arm

What did you feel?
   Sharp pain
      *(Rate it on a scale of 1–10, with ten being the
      most severe pain)*
   Dull pain *(Rate it 1–10 for severity)*
   Tingling *(Rate it 1–10 for severity)*
   Numbness *(Rate it 1–10 for severity)*
   Your hand/arm fell asleep

Have you felt it again since the first time?
   Does it feel the same? If different, how so?
   Has it spread to another area?

Do you feel it:
   Occasionally
   Regularly
   Constantly

Is there a pattern describing when the pain occurs?
When you are sleeping?
When you are working?
Another time?

How long does the pain last?

How often does the pain occur?

Does the pain get better or worse with activity?
What type of activity makes it better?
What type of activity makes it worse?

Overall, is the pain getting better, staying the same, or getting worse?

Has anyone else in your work place had similar sensations?

Has anyone else in your family had similar sensations?

Have you or anyone in your family had arthritis, lupus, or other diseases affecting the joints?

Have you ever been diagnosed with a CTD in the past?

YOUR WORK

What is your job?

Have any of your co-workers been diagnosed as having CTDs?

Does your job involve:
Repetitive motions
High levels of force
Awkward postures
Vibration
Direct pressure on or near the part of your hand/arm
where the symptoms occurred
Unvarying work positions
Stress

Does the repetitive motion involve:
Your fingers
Your hands
Your wrists
Your forearms
Your elbows
Your shoulders
Your neck

Do you use force:
Occasionally

Sometimes
Always

When you use force, are you:
Holding a tool
  A knife
  A hand tool (e.g., a screwdriver)
  A power tool
Holding an object
  With your fingers
  With your whole hand
Lifting objects
  With handles
  From the bottom
  Is the object hard to grasp?

Do your awkward postures involve:
Your fingers
  Spread fingers
  Bent fingers
  Detailed movements (e.g., screwing on a nut by hand in a tight space)
Your wrist
  Flexion (bent toward your palm)
  Extension (bent toward the back of your hand)
  Ulnar deviation (bent toward your little finger)
  Radial deviation (bent toward your thumb)
Your forearm:
  Pronation (turning so that your palm is down)
  Supination (turning so that your palm is up)
Your elbow:

Pronation
Supination
In combination with:
    Wrist extension
    Wrist flexion
Your shoulder:
    Arms above your head
    Reaching out in front of you
    Reaching behind you
    Reaching to the side

Is direct pressure produced by:
The edge of:
    Your work surface
    A keyboard
The arm of your chair
A tool (e.g., pliers)

Is the vibration caused by:
A pneumatic tool
A buffing machine
A grinding machine
Another power tool

Do you stay more or less in one position for:
An hour
Two hours
All day

If your job does not require that you move around, do you take rest breaks?

How often?

For how long?

Is your job stressful?

> **What is the cause of the stress?**
>   High production quotas
>   Unpredictable surges in work load
>   Cutbacks in personnel
>   Fear of losing your job
>   Poor supervision
>   Constant monitoring
>   Too little control over your job
>   Boredom
>   Conflicts with co-workers
>   Too little contact with co-workers
>   Poor working conditions

YOUR OWN DIAGNOSIS

Do you think you have developed a CTD? Which one? (See Chapter 7)

What do you think caused it?

How severe is it?

What do you think should be changed to prevent it in the future?

Have you discussed your condition with your employer?

When You See Your Doctor

The doctor's examination probably will consist of two parts—a medical/work history and a physical exam in which she does a series of simple tests similar to but more extensive than those described in Chapter 7. In some instances, depending on the physician, she may also use electrodiagnostic testing.

The Medical and Work History

Rely on the notes you prepared using the preceding outline. Try to keep your information succinct, since your doctor will be busy.

Your doctor is going to ask you questions that might rule out various diseases and ailments. For instance, she will probably ask you a series of questions to find out if there is a history of arthritis in your family. She is not asking these questions because she doubts that your condition is work-related but because they enable her to eliminate various ailments that have symptoms similar to those associated with CTDs.

She may also ask you to demonstrate what you do in your job. Though it may be difficult to mimic the actual positions you work in or the movements you do, try to be as accurate as possible. Be equally careful not to exaggerate. The more precisely you can inform your doctor, the better your chances are of an accurate diagnosis and helpful treatment.

Your doctor may be skeptical that you have a work-related condition. She may be right, or she may not be aware of the prevalence of CTDs and their association with job-related risk factors. Ask for clear explanations, as free of medical language as possible. Do not hesitate to make notes or to ask the doctor for a separate write-up of her reasons. This could prove helpful if you seek a second opinion.

Your Physical Exam

Your physician will likely start the exam by examining the area or areas where you have experienced pain, numbness, or other sensations. If she suspects a CTD, she is primarily interested in establishing four facts:

• *Is the illness a CTD?*

• *Where—exactly—is the CTD?* This is vital to proper treatment.

• *How severe is the CTD?* If the illness first produced symptoms only recently, it is more likely to respond to conservative (nonsurgical) treatment. This means your life will be disrupted minimally.

• *How long have you had the CTD?* It is often difficult to be precise, but together you might be able to identify an activity (at work or elsewhere) that can be associated with the type and location of your CTD. You can then estimate the date the illness started by when you started that activity.

The methods she uses to examine you will depend on the type of illness she suspects. Chapter 7 includes brief descriptions of the basic methods, though your doctor will do more involved tests in most cases.

Do not be surprised if the tests produce different sensations or responses in you than they did when you tried them at home. Be sure to tell your doctor if this happens. CTDs can produce good days and bad days. If, for example, your tendinitis is not acting up the day you are examined for whatever reason, it may be hard for the doctor to observe your symptoms.

Another factor to be considered is whether the exam is done on a Monday or after another prolonged break from work, in the evening right after work, or after you have been on leave from your job for medical or other reasons. For most CTDs, rest and time to recover are the best antidotes. This factor could influence your doctor's diagnosis of your condition. If possible, schedule your examination for the end of a working day when your symptoms will probably be easiest to observe.

Tell your doctor when you worked most recently or the last time you did the activity you suspect is responsible for your condition. Along the same lines, even if you have not worked in several days, try to recall whether you did any chores or tasks with your hands that might have affected your condition. Finally, if the day you are examined happens to be a "good" day or a "bad" day, make sure your doctor knows.

Electrodiagnostic tests

Doctors currently rely primarily on three different methods of electrodiagnostic testing—nerve conduction velocity (NCV), electromyography (EMG), and vibrometry. They use the tests for nerve-related illnesses such as carpal tunnel syndrome, ulnar nerve entrapment at the wrist or elbow, and thoracic outlet syndrome.

A small number of specialists also use X rays and magnetic resonance imaging (MRI) for diagnoses, but these tests are expensive and, for that reason, uncommon.

Nerve Conduction Velocity Testing

Your nerves conduct electrical signals. Nerve conduction velocity (NCV) testing—which Dr. Jeffrey Katz of Harvard Medical School in Boston has called the "diagnostic gold standard" for nerve-related CTDs—measures the speed at which the signal travels. A damaged nerve transmits the signal at a slower than normal speed.

If the results of your NCV test indicate nerve damage, it is likely—though not certain—that you have a relatively severe case that requires immediate attention and treatment. If your test does not indicate nerve damage, however, this does not put you in the clear.

NCV tests have a high threshold—that is, they usually detect nerve damage only when it has progressed significantly.

Because NCV tests can cost anywhere from $150 to $500, depending on where you live and the extent of the tests, and because they are of limited use, at best, for detecting nerve damage at early stages, they are used with restraint. Often, self-reporting of symptoms and simple, so-called provocative tests such as Phalen's test and Tinel's sign, are more sensitive, far less expensive, and therefore more practical (see page 181).

Electromyography

EMGs measure the responses of muscles to electrical stimuli, just as electrocardiograms (EKGs) measure the responses of heart muscles.

You have two kinds of nerves—those that carry sensory signals (allowing you to feel sensations) and those that carry motor signals (that move your muscles). EMGs are used to test the latter.

Even more than NCV tests, EMGs detect only advanced nerve damage. They are not generally useful in testing for CTDs involving tissue damage.

Vibrometry

A relatively new method of testing for nerve damage is vibrometry, in which multiple vibration frequencies are applied to one of the patient's fingers. The finger selected is one of those that gets its sensation from the nerve that is being tested.

The usefulness of vibrometry is not yet clear. Dr. Thomas Jetzer has found that although more study is needed, vibrometry could be a cost-effective tool for early detection of carpal tunnel syndrome because it is inexpensive (about $20 a test).

A research team headed by Dr. Francis Winn found vibrometry promising but cautioned that age, exposure to toxins, and other factors could produce insensitivities in the fingers like those caused by CTDs. This suggests that vibrometry should only be part of a broader diagnostic effort and that its stand-alone value is limited.

Getting a Diagnosis

Your physician will use all the information gathered to make a diagnosis and to prescribe treatment. Very likely, the doctor will decide one of four possible things:

• *Your symptoms do not indicate a CTD.* This could be because she considers your symptoms the signs of another condition, or because she does not believe that you are experiencing the symptoms you have reported.

• *You have a CTD and it is work-related.* Hopefully, she will also be able to identify the type of disorder. An accurate diagnosis is key to proper treatment, and it will prove helpful if you decide to pursue a claim for workers' compensation insurance or disability insurance.

• *You have a CTD but she cannot conclude that it is work-related.* This may make a workers' compensation or disability claim more difficult. The condition may have resulted from doing needlepoint, working in your wood shop, or some other activity.

• *You seem to have a CTD and she refers you to a specialist for more thorough testing and a more precise diagnosis.* This is most likely to happen for any of three reasons: She does not see many CTD cases and so feels unsure of the diagnosis, she is unsure what type of CTD you have (this is most common when there is more than one disorder present), or she believes the illness has progressed to a severe state and wants a specialist in CTDs to determine whether she is right or to provide specialized treatment. Of the three, the last is the most probable.

If possible, the doctor will tell you what type of CTD she thinks you have and where it appears to be located. She may also explain how severe, or advanced, the disorder is.

When the doctor gives you a diagnosis, do not be afraid to ask questions. Joan Lichterman says that she could have gotten better treatment if she had known more about CTDs before going to the doctor, told the doctor more about her working conditions, and asked more questions from the first visit on (see Chapter 1).

Many patients take a "doctor knows best" approach and accept what they are told, even when they have questions or doubts. This leaves them vulnerable to later feelings of anger if the treatment they receive is not effective.

You should take a different approach, one that has a more realistic view of how doctors work and that allows you to take an active role in your care. Even though your doctor knows more about health than you do, diagnoses rarely are clear-cut. This is particularly true with CTDs.

Your doctor makes her diagnosis on the basis of the symptoms you report, the likelihood that someone your age and gender and doing your job would develop a CTD, and the physical symptoms she is able to observe. Most of the time, this produces an accurate diagnosis. Even a slightly inaccurate diagnosis can lead to treatment that can help you get well because the treatments for many CTDs are similar.

Doctors are trained to make decisions quickly, so do not think that an immediate diagnosis is just a snap judgment. If you ask clear questions, your doctor will be able to explain why she made the diagnosis she did, how she ruled out other possible conditions, and what she thinks will be accomplished by what she has prescribed.

Sometimes the doctor's diagnosis does not accurately describe your condition and the prescribed treatment is not effective. You must then report back to your doctor, telling her what you experienced during the treatment as well as any new information you can provide. You might find it helpful to review the series of questions outlined on pages 114–121 before returning to your doctor.

Getting the Right Treatment

Just as many doctors disagree about the diagnosis of CTDs, there is a spectrum of opinion about the best way to treat them. Generally, the standard course of treatment is to begin with the least disruptive and least expensive options, proceeding as necessary to the more involved ones. This means starting with *conservative* treatments, going next to *medical* treatments, and using *surgical* treatments only in the most extreme cases.

Conservative Treatments

The primary purpose of conservative treatments is to allow the ailing tissue or nerve to heal itself. For CTDs involving the hand and wrist, many doctors prescribe a *splint* to immobilize the injured area and allow it to recover. The splints are either worn all day (for tendinitis and tenosynovitis) or at night (for carpal tunnel syndrome and other nerve-related disorders).

For tendinitis and tenosynovitis, the most common type of splint is a "cock-up" splint that immobilizes your wrist in a slightly extended (bending toward the back of your hand) posture. These can be found in almost any drugstore.

On occasion, particularly if the disorder resulted from repeated wrist extension, a cock-up splint may prove painful. A flatter splint to keep the wrist in a neutral position might be better.

The flatter splint is most often used to immobilize

wrists in which carpal tunnel sydrome and ulnar nerve compression at the wrist have developed. By maintaining the wrist in a neutral position, the flatter splint allows the opening of the carpal tunnel and the passageway for the ulnar nerve (Guyon's tunnel) to remain as large as possible.

Both types of splints consist of an inflexible, molded piece that wraps around the palm side of your hand and wrist and is held firmly in place by elastic straps that wrap around your wrist.

Another type of splint for carpal tunnel syndrome consists of a stiff, straight piece that rests against the back side of your lower forearm and hand. Elastic straps at both ends effectively immobilize your wrist but allow you considerable freedom of movement with your hand and fingers, an advantage over other splints. This is a relatively new approach but many people with carpal tunnel syndrome who have tried it report that it seems to work well.

When the CTD is in the shoulder, a shoulder sling is often used. This serves the same function as splints, restricting movement.

Whenever immobilization is used, there are three things to be concerned about. First, your muscles may lose their tone. This is usually not serious if the period of immobilization is just a few weeks, since you will regain muscle tone quickly with exercise. Second, joints can become stiff and lose mobility. This, too, usually can be overcome quickly with exercise. Finally, anyone wearing a splint and trying to continue to do his job can instead aggravate his condition.

Hot and cold compresses are sometimes used as part of a conservative treatment. Cold should be applied soon after swelling occurs to reduce the swelling and to allow as much mobility as possible in the affected area.

Heat can increase blood flow in soft tissue such as muscles and tendons, aiding healing and reducing pain or discomfort. If an area is swollen, heat should be avoided, since increased blood flow can add to the swelling.

Do not use heat or cold compresses if you have, or suspect you have, a nerve-related illness. Increasing the mobility of your wrist in the case of carpal tunnel syndrome could lead to further damage.

Exercise and *physical therapy* are useful only after your condition has been stabilized and the injured tissue is recovering. Even then, they should be done only under supervision of a physical therapist or another health professional. Often exercises are not recommended for hand and wrist CTDs. When your CTD involves nerve damage, only do exercises prescribed by your doctor.

Generally, exercises stretch your muscles and tendons, improve blood circulation, reduce muscle tension, and improve joint motion. They are always a good idea as a preventive measure before you start work and periodically through the working day. See page 61 for more on exercises.

Physical therapy is a licensed profession that requires extensive medical and clinical training. There are more than forty thousand physical therapists in the

United States, and their training qualifies them to work with CTD patients. They can help refine a diagnosis, set realistic treatment and rehabilitation goals, deliver treatment, and help identify potential CTD causes. Some physical therapists also are qualified to recommend on-the-job CTD prevention methods.

Lucy Jacobs, a physical therapist in Fresno, California, who is known for her work with CTD patients, gets most of her referrals from physicians. The first thing she does with new patients is evaluate their strength, mobility, degree of pain, and swelling. She also tries to assess what they can and cannot do. Occasionally, she visits a patient's workplace to evaluate possible causes and, if appropriate, to suggest changes.

The first step in treatment is a two-week rest period, for which she usually prescribes a custom splint or sling to immobilize the affected area. In addition, if the patient's physician prescribed anti-inflammatory medication, she makes sure that he is taking it. Most people believe they only need to take the medication if they are feeling acute pain, she says.

After the rest period, she uses massage to stimulate the muscles and to separate scar tissue from muscle tissue. She often also uses heat, stretching exercises, and a vibrator to encourage muscle and tendon flexibility. In most cases, she shows the patient a series of gentle exercises he can do at home for several weeks.

She expects most patients to experience decreased pain within two weeks of first seeing her. If after four weeks the patient's pain has not abated at all, she refers him back to the doctor for a more through medical evaluation.

The Alexander Technique and The Feldenkrais Method:

People with CTDs who do not want to rely solely on physical therapy, standard medical care, or other conventional treatment methods can explore options such as the Alexander Technique and the Feldenkreis Method.

The Alexander Technique developed from the principle that we all learn habits of improper "use" of our bodies that adversely affect our health, and that we can teach ourselves how to unlearn them. These habits develop constantly in both small and large ways—ranging from grinding your teeth to clenching the muscles in your lower back when you experience stress.

The Alexander Technique teaches you to observe your movement and tension patterns and habits, to become aware of how they may be interfering with your use, and to learn how to use less effort in your work.

The Alexander Technique helped me to resolve carpal tunnel syndrome in both wrists and to return to working at a computer. (In addition to the Alexander Technique, my treatment for carpal tunnel syndrome involved rest—I rarely touched a computer keyboard for about one year.) I took one fifty-minute lesson per week for about eighteen months and practiced the technique constantly the rest of the time. Within a few months, the symptoms of carpal tunnel syndrome were gone. Though I am no longer taking lessons, I still use the technique daily.

Lessons involved no massage or stretching. Instead, my instructor gave light physical guidance and verbal instructions to make me aware of my habits and to remind me how to move (or not move) without engaging my counterproductive habits.

The Feldenkrais Method was developed by a man who had studied the Alexander Technique and other body work methods. Its goal is to give you the ability to move with a minimum of energy, tension, and friction—in short, in the most efficient way possible.

Richard Adelman, a Feldenkrais instructor based in Berkeley, California, says that the method can reduce uneven movements that can contribute to CTDs. For example, computer users who move with jerky movements—even very slight jerkiness—can significantly increase the amount of force with which they strike keyboard keys. In effect, this creates a CTD risk where one need not be.

Both the Alexander Technique and the Feldenkrais Method are popular among musicians and actors seeking to make maximum use of their bodies. They also are gaining a following among athletes and the general public. They can be helpful to people with CTDs. There are many other non-medical models, of course, and you may want to explore them.

To learn more about the two methods, use the following contact information to find out if there is an instructor in your area:

• North American Society of Teachers of the Alexander Technique, PO Box 3992, Champaign, IL 61826, (217) 359-3529.

• The Feldenkrais Guild, 524 Ellsworth Street, Albany, OR 97321, (503) 926-0981.

Medical Treatments

Many doctors prescribe medicine for CTDs and consider medical treatment a type of conservative treatment. All three of the medical treatments that follow are used primarily to reduce inflammation to allow damaged tissue to heal.

Aspirin and ibuprofen often are recommended because both reduce swelling of inflamed tissue and relieve pain. In addition, they are inexpensive and readily available. For many CTD cases, immobilization, rest, and one of these anti-inflammatory painkillers is sufficient for full recovery. Ibuprofen is a nonprescription type of *nonsteroidal anti-inflammatory drug* (NSAID).

Corticosteroids can be injected directly into inflamed tendons and bursa. Because the drug is delivered directly to the site, it can produce dramatically quick and significant reductions in swelling, often within forty-eight hours. Some patients initially feel worse, but most feel better quickly.

Success depends primarily on accurate location of the damaged tissue. The flip side of delivering the corticosteroid (cortisone is one type) locally is that a misplaced injection is of little use, while repeated injections can cause the tendon to rupture. In addition, some physicians believe that cortisteroids can ultimately slow the healing process.

Other doctors use these injections as their primary means of treatment. Says one doctor who regularly treats people who have developed CTDs in the poultry processing industry, "If you tell them to wear splints, a lot of people will forget. If you tell them not to go back to their jobs, they'll tell you that they can't afford not to. If you tell them to take aspirin or you prescribe an anti-inflammatory drug, they'll take them for a few days, stop feeling pain, and stop taking the pills. With cortisone injections, I can make sure the medication gets to the problem."

Surgical Treatments

Surgery for tendinitis and tenosynovitis is rare but not unheard of. In almost all cases, persistent treatment by conservative or medical methods are more effective and less risky.

Nerve-related CTDs can be quite another story. Some advanced cases of carpal tunnel syndrome, in particular, as well as ulnar nerve entrapments at the wrist and at the elbow and thoracic outlet syndrome, must be treated surgically or the nerve damage will continue to worsen.

What is most difficult is deciding when surgery must be done.* Many hand surgeons recommend carpal tunnel release surgery without hesitation. As operations go, it is simple, the risks of complications are small, and the chances of success are good. There

---

*This discussion will focus on surgery for carpal tunnel syndrome. It is believed to be the most common surgery performed under the workers' compensation system, according to Dr. Paul Cotton, with as many as three hundred thousand carpal tunnel release procedures performed annually. Surgery is less common for the other nerve-related disorders.

is some concern that the long-term results of carpal tunnel surgery may be less than glowing, however.

The objective of carpal tunnel surgery, or carpal tunnel release, is to sever the carpal ligament, a tough connective tissue that crosses the wrist at the base of the hand. (It is known medically as the *flexor retinaculum*.) The primary purpose of the ligament is to hold in place the tendons that pass through the wrist's carpal tunnel along with the median nerve. Since carpal tunnel syndrome is the result of compression of the median nerve by the tendons, it seems logical to relieve pressure on the nerve by effectively unbanding the area.

The traditional surgical method in use for more than four decades is known as *open carpal tunnel surgery*. An incision of about two inches is made through the skin covering the carpal ligament. The ligament is then severed.

More recently, several surgeons have developed a "closed" method that requires a smaller incision across the forearm near the base of the hand. A special scalpel is inserted through the incision and used to sever the ligament.

One of the leading proponents of the closed method, Dr. David Pagnanelli of Abington, Pennsylvania, says that recovery from this method of surgery is considerably quicker than it is from open surgery. While open surgery often keeps the patient from returning to work for up to several months, Pagnanelli reports that about half of 251 closed surgery patients returned to work within one week of the surgery and nearly three-quarters returned to work within three weeks.

Like all surgery, carpal tunnel release surgery involves risks. The most significant is the danger that the median nerve itself can be nicked or cut during either type of surgery, causing permanent damage.

In addition, a high number of people who have carpal tunnel release surgery find that their symptoms recur though usually not as severely as they originally occurred. A study done by a team at the State University of New York at Buffalo found that "57 per cent of the cases had return of some symptom beginning after an average of two years. . . . Most often these symptoms are not significant enough to prompt the patient to again seek medical treatment."

Ultimately, the best treatment for job-related CTDs of all kinds may be identifying the factors that caused the disorder and then correcting them. When that cannot be done, the choice may be between your job and your health. Warns NIOSH's Vern Putz-Anderson, "if a complete and permanent recovery is expected, it is important the *worker is not returned to the same job or task that precipitated the CTD*" (emphasis in original).

After You See Your Doctor

Once you have developed a CTD, you may have to make several important decisions. The first is whether to file for workers' compensation or disability insurance.

Workers' compensation insurance is intended to cover all medical costs if you are injured or made ill at work. Workers' compensation also reimburses you for a share of your wages. The insurance premiums are paid by your employer. The workers' compensation system has a flip side, as well, in that it prohibits employees from suing their employers for work-related health problems. If you feel your employer is or should be responsible for your illness, you must rely on the workers' compensation system.

Every state handles workers' compensation in its own way, so you will probably need to consult either a union representative, if you belong to a union, or a lawyer, or both.

Experiences with workers' compensation can vary widely. Caroline Rose, an editor whose experience with CTDs led her to form a network of people with CTDs in the San Francisco area, says that her doctor had immediately diagnosed her as having work-related tendinitis. "I never had trouble on the workers' compensation end," she explains. Others who have had their claims for compensation contested have struggled for years before receiving compensation.

CTDs cost workers' compensation insurance companies $20 billion or more a year, according to estimates made by Aetna Life and Casualty, one of the nation's largest insurance companies.

Disability insurance can partially make up for lost wages while you are unable to work due to a CTD condition. Not all states currently require employers to carry disability insurance, however. If you work in a state without mandatory insurance—a lawyer can tell you whether you do—and your work presents a high risk for CTDs, you can consider taking out a personal disability insurance policy.

When you are ready to return to work, you may want to arrange with your employer to go to a new job that does not involve the activities that you believe caused your CTD. Even if your employer is willing to help you, this may prove difficult in some industries. If you are a data entry clerk by training, you may find it difficult to identify a job that does not put you at risk. On the other hand, you may be able to negotiate placement in a position that represents a career move.

The 1990 Americans with Disabilities Act may help many people disabled by CTDs return to work. Because the law is new, however, it is not yet possible to know how broad its effect will be.

The disabilities act was developed to protect disabled workers from discrimination. It requires that as long as a disabled worker is able to perform the "essential elements" of a job, employers must make reasonable accommodations for the person.

This means that a computer user with a CTD could be entitled to a voice-driven computer system that virtually eliminates the need for a keyboard, or that an auto mechanic could request and receive reassignment to a counter service job.

As with workers' compensation and disability insurance, you may need to consult with a lawyer for help with the Americans with Disabilities Act.

Outside of work you should make smart, healthy decisions for yourself. For instance, if you are a bowler and you have experienced a wrist or hand CTD, you probably should forgo bowling. If you like to play tennis but your CTD is tennis elbow, you may want to find a new sport or at least take lessons to correct your technique. If you love needlework but are recovering from carpal tunnel release surgery, it is time to develop a new craft skill.

Do not assume that because your condition has been resolved you are now back to your old self. Many CTDs can leave you permanently vulnerable to recurring disorders. Only you can make the decisions about which activities you can resume safely and which are out of bounds for you.

CHAPTER 5

Is There a CTD Epidemic?

It is easy to label the rise in the number of new CTD cases over the past fifteen years an epidemic (see Table 5.1), but it is considerably more difficult to say with confidence what that means.

One school of thought contends that the reported rise includes only a relatively small number of new CTD cases. The balance of the reported cases is the result of a mix of media-generated panic, misdiagnoses, and marketing hype by companies seeking to capitalize on people's fears.

Another view is that the epidemic comprises not only new cases brought on by steady increases in computerization and automation but also includes cases that were not counted in the past. This is a result of increased awareness among workers, better diagnoses by physicians, and more attention to CTDs in general by OSHA.

Dr. Larry Fine, one of the top occupational health specialists in the federal government, believes that there is an epidemic but that it is not simply explained. "A lot of it is increased awareness. Workers and doctors are more aware. There have been changes in the techniques of work, and they contribute to this problem. There have probably also been changes in the work force that are part of it. Better record keeping is undoubtedly a part of it."

TABLE 5.1
Reported CTD Cases by Year: 1978–1991

Year	Number of cases	Percent of all Nerve-Related Illnesses
1978	20,200	14%
1979	21,900	15%
1980	23,200	18%
1981	23,000	18%
1982	22,600	21%
1983	26,700	25%
1984	37,700	28%
1985	37,000	30%
1986	45,500	33%
1987	72,900	38%
1988	115,300	48%
1989	146,900	52%
1990	185,400	56%
1991	223,600	61%

Source: Bureau of Labor Statistics. These statistics are based on the number of new cases of CTDs reported by private U.S. companies to OSHA. Public employers, most notably the U.S. Postal Service, are not counted here. The Postal Service is the largest nondefense employer in the United States and CTD rates in some occupations there have consistently occurred in more than 20 percent of the workers.

The Question of Undercounting

Labor union representatives are certain that the problem is far worse than the federal statistics indicate. In a July 31, 1991, letter to then-Secretary of Labor Lynn Martin, a coalition of labor unions seeking an emergency ergonomics standard argued that the increase "is the result of more than just better reporting." The unions spotlight "real and substantial" workplace changes such as computer terminals and other new technology, increased work pace, and the reduction of jobs to "smaller, more repetitive tasks."

They contend that research shows that the BLS data reported in Table 5.1 significantly undercount the rate of all CTDs: "These studies indicate that the actual rates of work-related cumulative trauma disorders are actually 50 to 100 times greater than rates reported" by the BLS.

The unions are suggesting that the number of new work-related CTDs for 1991, the latest year for which data are available, was between 11 million and 22 million. These numbers are staggering, particularly considering that the total number of reported occupational illnesses (including CTDs) reported in 1991 was less than 500,000 and the total work force was about 130 million.

The chances that so many workers have developed CTDs seem remote, but not out of the question. Vern Putz-Anderson of NIOSH and other occupational health specialists agree that more than half of the American work force can be considered at risk. Meanwhile, studies consistently have found that about 20 percent of workers in high-risk industries develop CTDs. Simple mathematics affirms that 10 million to 15 million new cases a year is not unthinkable (130 million workers times 50 percent = 65 million; times 20 percent = 13 million). Since not all industries involve high-risk work, however, the actual number is lower than this. How much lower we cannot know.

Undercounting on the scale proposed by the unions also is suggested by a study done by the California Occupational Health Program (COHP). This investigation surveyed health care practitioners in Santa Clara County, to gauge the occurrence of carpal tunnel syndrome there. Just 30 percent of the 1,698 doctors contacted by COHP responded, reporting 7,214 patients treated for carpal tunnel syndrome in 1987. Of these, 3,413 cases were identified as work-related.

In 1987, Santa Clara County physicians also were required to report all suspected occupational illnesses to the state. Remarkably, just 71 cases were reported, or about 2 percent of the 3,413 cases found by COHP according to the federal Centers for Disease Control. This difference is consistent with the undercounting figure posed by the labor unions.

Why the Data Are Inaccurate

Officials at BLS, which is part of the Department of Labor, recognize that their methods of counting occupational illnesses do not reliably count CTDs. BLS draws its numbers from information submitted to OSHA by private employers. Public employers such as the U.S. Postal Service, as well as state and local government, are not counted.

This system was developed initially for counting occupational injuries and generally is not considered appropriate for occupational illnesses. Because CTDs and other illnesses develop gradually, they often are not easily attributed to work-related causes. Injuries on the job are rarely overlooked, by comparison.*

In addition, CTDs of the arms and hands are lumped together with other occupational illnesses resulting from cumulative causes such as lower back pain and hearing loss. Indeed, though the figures listed in Table 5.1 are widely cited for CTDs involving only the arm and hand, they actually include other types of CTDs, including hearing loss due to prolonged noise exposure. This means that we can only guess how prevalent arm and hand CTDs are.

In fact, NIOSH officials warn that currently there is no way to use existing data bases to accurately estimate the frequency of CTDs and their cost to the country.

For years BLS officials have discussed ways to improve the bureau's counting of job-related illnesses. In late 1992 they floated a proposal to base their statistics not solely on disorders that were diagnosed by physicians and reported by companies but to also use other data, such as lost work time. In addition, BLS is

---

BLS calls ailments that were caused by a single incident, such as falling off a ladder, injuries, while those resulting from chronic or cumulative causes are illnesses.

proposing to collect information about the type of equipment being used that could help to improve understanding of CTDs and other occupational health issues. These changes would likely improve the value of the data.

Officials at OSHA also are discussing ways of revising their data collection methods. At the earliest, these methods would be used for data collected in 1992 and released in early 1994. And even the top ergonomist at OSHA is wary of how the new methods will work. "Theoretically, the new guidelines are supposed to make the situation better, but who knows what it will look like when we actually get through with it?" Dr. Roger Stephens told *VDT News*.

Calculating CTD Costs

Without better statistics, we cannot know what CTDs have cost and what they will cost. Insurance companies, which most often end up paying the bills associated with occupational illnesses, ranging from medical care to workers' compensation, have the most immediate reason to know.

In 1984, when the number of CTDs reported to BLS totaled about 17 percent of the number in 1991, the American Academy of Orthopedic Surgeons estimated that lost earnings and the costs of medical care for CTDs exceeded $27 billion per year. More recently, the National Council on Compensation Insurance has placed the average cost of a diagnosed CTD case at $29,000. Using the BLS figures for 1991, this puts the total direct costs at about $6.5 billion. If you accept the adjustment of fifty or a hundred times higher that the unions have suggested, the annual costs dwarf anything now being discussed.

In 1991, Aetna Casualty and Surety, one of the nation's largest insurance companies, estimated that CTDs cost American employers about $20 billion a year in workers' compensation–related costs. Aetna found that about 45 percent of the workers' compensation claims and some 63 percent of the claim payments it handled at several large companies were for CTDs. Aetna's figure is widely used, but Aetna emphasizes that the figure was estimated using crude methods and that the company never meant for it to be more than a rough approximation.

In addition, because this figure does not factor in the costs of CTDs not covered by workers' compensation, such as medical care provided outside of the workers' compensation system—and there is every reason to believe that these costs are substantial—$20 billion may be significantly below the real total cost.

Statistics and Prevention

Which figure is correct? Unfortunately, we do not know. This lack of knowledge limits our efforts to develop policies for preventing CTDs. It also mutes any incentive and justification the data might provide to pursue new research.

For an effective prevention policy, we need data that are not only reliable but also comprehensive. The hundreds of scientific research papers that have been published describing CTDs and their causes have given us a general understanding of the problem, but have not resolved many controversies about causes, diagnoses, and treatment.

As difficult as good studies may be to complete, the federal government or the insurance companies, or the two together, are eventually going to have to find the funds to pay for the type of long-term studies that will markedly improve the diagnosis, treatment, and, most important, prevention of CTDs. These studies would follow large numbers of workers at risk for CTDs over a long period and would evaluate psychosocial as well as physical risk factors. If you want to develop an effective prevention scheme, you really have to understand how all of these factors interact, says NIOSH's Dr. Larry Fine.

As long as we allow ourselves to remain uncertain whether an epidemic is occurring, that research will not be done. While NIOSH is required by law to continue conducting health hazard evaluations of workplaces thought to pose a hazard, the agency is not planning to undertake this sort of major, expensive new research. This does not mean that preventive efforts based on our current understanding cannot be effective, Fine adds. Indeed, he believes that we are near the peak of the CTD epidemic and that better awareness of causes, prevention, and treatment will cause the rate of new cases to decline.

CHAPTER 6

CTD Standards

While it is not always easy to decide how best to protect your own health and safety on the job, each individual case is much simpler than the task facing policymakers.

How do you set mandatory standards for all workers or even for a single industry that permit the high degree of flexibility that is central to ergonomic solutions? How do you account for variations among jobs and occupations without making the cost of implementing your standard excessive? How do you control physical and psychosocial factors that you do not understand as well as you would like to? These are just a few of the thorny questions confounding various government and private sector attempts to develop a workable and effective policy for reducing the number of CTDs.

Complicating the problem further is the lack of scientific data to determine the precise levels of force, repetition, and other CTD-associated risk factors that are safe. Clearly these factors are linked to CTDs, but people and jobs vary so much that researchers cannot say what is a safe level.

The increasing attention on psychosocial risk factors makes setting standards more difficult still. No research tells us how important psychosocial factors are relative to physical ones. More important, that research will not be done anytime soon. A study tracking the health of a large number of workers (one thousand or more) over several years and evaluating both their physical and psychosocial working conditions could resolve many questions. NIOSH's Dr. Lawrence Fine calls it the logical next step.

But the complexity and the cost of such a project are prohibitive, given limited research funds. NIOSH is the only federal agency currently supporting CTD research and the ergonomics furniture industry is not supporting new research on this scale. As a result, the data that could resolve many important questions will not be available to help current standard-setting attempts. In fact, even if the "logical" study were started in 1993, results would not be available until at least 1998, according to Fine.

Fine says that whatever standards are developed will have to rely on the available, limited research data. "We are going to be dealing with the CTD problem with our current level of understanding for some time," he says.

How, then, to shape a CTD safety policy?

In addition to the day-to-day policy-making that goes on in workplaces everywhere, there are a small number of coordinated efforts under way to set standards to reduce the number of CTDs. Potentially the most important one is being undertaken by OSHA. The state of California also is working on a mandatory standard, and several independent, industry-led efforts are attempting to establish voluntary guidelines.

What follows is a description of these developments.

OSHA

On August 3, 1992, OSHA published an advanced notice of public rulemaking (ANPR)—the first official step toward a federal CTD standard—asking businesses, trade associations, labor unions, doctors, public health specialists, individuals, and others for their comments on the idea. The ANPR consisted of a description of research results and a series of questions regarding the need for and potential scope of a standard.

It suggested that OSHA's ergonomics specialists are considering a broad definition of ergonomics that would include both physical and psychosocial factors and a standard that covers all occupations rather than just high-risk ones such as meat cutting and computer work.

Clearly, they believe that the rapid rise in CTD cases over the past fifteen years coupled with the now-epidemic rates has to be addressed by the federal government. "The increasing number of ergonomic disorders affecting employees in a wide variety of industries and the significant costs of these disorders to employees, employers, and society suggest that a regulation to prevent, eliminate, and reduce ergonomic hazards in the work place may be necessary," the agency concludes in its ANPR. OSHA's options include a mandatory standard, a policy guidance document that would allow employers to set their own policies, and an aggressive federal training and education program that does not rely on standards or a guidance. Of course, OSHA could also decide to do nothing.

In the absence of clear federal direction on CTDs, the courts are starting to play a role in shaping CTD policy. At the same time, action by OSHA could influence the outcomes of lawsuits. The mere existence of an OSHA standard would make it easier for people with CTDs to win lawsuits by creating the presumption that CTDs are recognized occupational hazards. If OSHA eventually decided that a CTD standard is not justified, that decision, too, will influence the outcome of suits. At the same time, a series of successful suits by people with CTDs against either their employers or equipment manufacturers would put pressure on OSHA (and state occupational health agencies) to enact a standard that could bring order to a complicated legal situation.

More than 210 individuals and organizations responded to the ANPR, and the comments were widely divergent. While labor unions argued forcefully for a final standard as quickly as possible, most business and industry respondents countered that ambiguities in the research data make a standard not only unjustifiable but also impossible to enforce. The Center for Office Technology (COT), a coalition of twenty-five major computer makers and users including Apple Computer, AT&T, and IBM Corporation, said that "there is not reliable medical research on which to form a health-based standard."

This reasoning raises the critical question of cause-and-effect—that is, if you cannot clearly establish a cause-and-effect link between a suspected risk factor and CTDs, how can you regulate a solution? As with other occupational health issues, how OSHA views this question will determine whether a standard gets developed and, if so, what it will cover.

Scientists have strict but not absolute rules for determining when a cause-and-effect relationship exists. COT, in its comments to OSHA, is urging OSHA to use a scientific standard to determine policy.

Occupational health policy-making often requires judgments—usually controversial ones, however. Even many occupational risk factors that already are strictly regulated, such as asbestos and many toxic chemicals, have not been shown to be linked to illness, in some scientists' minds. Yet rejecting safeguards against asbestos or toxics is widely considered bad policy.

As OSHA proceeds in its rulemaking process, it will have to resolve the cause-and-effect question and many other sharply contested issues, including:

• How reliable are the Bureau of Labor Statistics' annual count of CTDs? While labor representatives believe that the BLS data significantly understate the extent of the problem, many industry comments on OSHA's ANPR suggested that CTD problem is not as severe as media coverage of the BLS reports suggest.

• Should OSHA develop a mandatory standard (labor's view)? Or should CTD issues be worked out between management and labor?

• Are the costs of CTD treatment, including workers' compensation and other insurance costs, greater than the costs of prevention, as labor groups contend? Industry argues that the costs of implementing an OSHA standard would be substantial and, given the scientific uncertainty, unjustified.

• What role should psychosocial factors associated with CTDs play in a standard? Labor advocates say that since the purpose of the standard is to prevent CTDs, all factors—including psychosocial ones—should be covered. Businesses follow two different approaches. The first is that the emphasis on psychosocial factors shows that there is too much scientific uncertainty to proceed with a standard. The second is that psychosocial factors plainly fall outside of OSHA's jurisdiction and should not, under any circumstances, be included in a standard.

• Is more research needed? Both sides of the debate agree that it is. Labor would like to have more precise information to guide prevention strategies, while industry believes that a thorough research effort would prove that CTDs are not linked in a significant way to work.

• Are public hearings necessary for OSHA to learn more about the extent and nature of the CTD epidemic? Because labor unions want fast action, they argue against public hearings. Industry groups, determined to slow what they consider a misguided OSHA initiative, favor hearings.

Taken together, the ANPR comments do very little to resolve the question of whether to develop a standard. In any event, no standard is likely before 1996. Even if OSHA moves quickly from the ANPR to a notice of proposed rulemaking, the next step in federal standard-setting protocol, that notice would be subject to the same type of comment period that the ANPR was. Likewise for any subsequent proposed rulemaking before a final rule, or standard, can be issued.

Absent a standard, OSHA must rely on its general authority to protect worker safety and health to attempt to prevent CTDs. Unfortunately, this approach has proved uneven, at best. Despite several highly publicized multimillion-dollar fines in the late 1980s and early 1990s against employers for serious CTD-related problems, OSHA officials concede that the agency's enforcement is limited to spot-checking. At a 1991 congressional hearing, OSHA officials said that the agency had just four people on staff assigned specifically to CTD safety.

California's Efforts to Enact a CTD Standard

In 1989, after two years of study, an ad hoc video display terminal (VDT) advisory committee to the California Occupational Safety and Health Administration (CalOSHA) urged CalOSHA to develop regulations for computer users and to include CTD risk factors in the rules. CalOSHA officials rejected the recommendation and instead opted to begin work on a CTD standard for workers in all industries.

In a series of tense meetings over the next three years, representatives from CalOSHA, business groups, and labor unions negotiated what the standard should cover, how it should be enforced, and how extensive its provisions would be.

On June 1, 1992, CalOSHA issued a draft standard for public comment that neither the labor groups nor the business representatives supported. It sought to encourage employees to report CTDs and specified four possible conditions that could trigger a CalOSHA work site evaluation. The first possible trigger would be an employee report of one or more CTD symptoms, a provision demanded by labor officials who feared that too few evaluations would be done if CalOSHA waited for employers to report CTD problems. In addition, the draft standard called for training of all workers, instead of just high-risk workers, as business groups had urged.

Because of these provisions, a coalition of business leaders concluded that they could not support the standard, casting doubt on CalOSHA's ability to issue it in a final form. Labor groups also were withholding support. A CalOSHA spokesman said that the agency was considering various options, including tacking the CTD rules onto an existing regulation on job safety.

By early 1993, several months after the CTD standard was supposed to be presented to CalOSHA's standards board and just as federal OSHA officials were reviewing the comments submitted in response to their ANPR, the proposal remained in limbo. CalOSHA officials conceded that they could not effectively implement the standard as long as business leaders oppose it.

Federal OSHA officials, aware of the sharp disagreements between business and labor representatives in the agency's ANPR comments, no doubt took note of the California experience. If OSHA proceeds with its CTD standard, will it fare better than CalOSHA has so far?

Voluntary Guidelines

The American National Standards Institute (ANSI) is a national clearinghouse for voluntary guidelines in a wide range of industries and for diverse purposes. Under its auspices in 1983, a panel of ergonomists began work on what would eventually become ANSI/HFS 100-1988, a VDT ergonomics guideline. With a minimum of controversy, the panel produced a technical document that included specifications for seating, keyboard setup, adjustable workstations, and other CTD-related factors. The standard, which is voluntary, was approved by ANSI in early 1988.

Under ANSI rules, the guideline must be revised within five years or it loses its ANSI seal of approval. The revision process started in 1992 and should be completed in 1994.

As the revision process started, a major concern about the 1988 guideline was its lack of attention to CTD-related factors. Rani Leuder, an ergonomics consultant with Humanics in Encino, California detailed the document's shortcoming in an analysis that was first published in *VDT News*. "The guidelines for keyboard design were developed before attention in the U.S. focused on [CTDs]. Ironically, these guidelines are now being used to try to prevent injuries that were poorly understood or ignored during the standard's development," Leuder wrote.

The group working on the revisions has divided into subcommittees to consider specific portions of the guideline. In addition to input devices such as mice, trackballs, and pens that were not included in the 1988 version, the revisions process will evaluate guidelines for workstation design. It is not expected to weigh psychosocial factors, however.

The State of New Jersey adopted sweeping voluntary guidelines in 1990 that include keyboard provisions drawn from the ANSI/HFS 100-1988 document, as well as periodic rest breaks and job rotation. Workers with CTD-related symptoms should be allowed to take additional, discretionary rest breaks, the guideline recommends.

A second ANSI panel is drafting a CTD guideline for all industries. Convened by the National Safety Council, the group is headed by Dr. Thomas Armstrong of the University of Michigan at Ann Arbor, who is one of the deans of the CTD field. The panel, ANSI Z365—Standards Committee on Control of Cumulative Trauma Disorders, is not expected to produce its guidelines before 1995.

Related Activity: Legislation and Lawsuits

Many states and municipalities have debated legislation to address working conditions for computers users, such as CTDs. Two localities—Suffolk County, New York and San Francisco—have enacted moderately tough laws, but the courts have ruled both statutes unenforceable. In both cases, business-backed legal challenges led the courts to rule that state occupational safety laws preempted the local governments' authority to enforce separate rules.

The CTD debate has also moved into the courts, where CTD policy is being shaped on a case-by-case basis. In the absence of a clear federal policy, many people with CTDs are finding that suing equipment manufacturers is the most effective way to gain compensation for the harm they believe they have suffered.

The CTD product liability suit is a boom business, particularly among computer operators. More than 250 CTD-related claims naming some 40 different companies were pending in one federal court alone in early 1993. The defendants include manufacturers of keyboards, computers, and grocery store scanners. In addition, one Communications Workers of America union local reported at about the same time that it was preparing more than 100 additional claims out of 650 reported CTD cases among its members.

In a related type of lawsuit, a Washington State woman who had sued Boeing Company for refusing to accommodate her request for a job reassignment after she developed a CTD was awarded $1.2 million. Janice Goodman had worked at a microfilm camera for almost five years when she went on disability leave in 1989. She contended that she had given her supervisor a note from her doctor stating that a job change was necessary but that the company rejected the request. Goodman sued under the state's antidiscrimination laws.

Lawsuits are emerging as a driving force behind CTD safety policy in the United States. Partly as a result, effective standards for controlling CTDs will be achieved only in bits and pieces, if at all. Though they are a problem of considerable medical and economic importance—perhaps *because* they are of considerable medical and economic importance—CTDs are likely to remain in political and scientific limbo for the foreseeable future. Until a clear and comprehensive policy is enacted, the most effective way to address CTDs in your life and on your job will continue to be following the suggestions in this book.

CHAPTER 7

Do You Have a CTD?
Symptoms and Screening Tests

Everyone has occasional aches and pains that are not cause for concern. The time to pay special attention to a pain is when it seems out of the ordinary or when it recurs. If your job involves repetition or awkward postures, the use of lots of muscular force, very little time for rest and recuperation, or a lot of stress, you should be on the watch for symptoms of cumulative trauma disorders.

If you experience strong or recurring aches and pains, keep a log of when you feel an unusual twinge of discomfort, tingling, or pain, or of when you experience numbness.

Your observations can be critical to an accurate diagnosis and proper treatment. While some CTDs are relatively easy to diagnose, others are not. Your doctor will make the initial diagnosis largely on the basis of your description. If you report only some of your symptoms, she may be misled into a partial diagnosis that could lead to inadequate or improper treatment.

Getting a proper diagnosis is essential. In addition to determining how to treat your CTD, the diagnosis may affect your claim for workers' compensation or for disability insurance if you file. It could influence how you discuss your condition with your boss or employer, or whether you discuss it at all. Finally, it could be important to researchers who want to know whether the treatment you receive is effective.

Getting an *early* diagnosis is also key, and you are the only person who will be aware of the initial signs of illness. You know your working conditions, your habits, and your symptoms better than anyone else does. Using self-reported symptoms to identify CTDs in their early stages is an effective screening tool, according to Vern Putz-Anderson, who has spent much of the last eighteen years studying CTDs at NIOSH. "We may see more cases but decreased severity. Ultimately, that's a good thing," he explains. The earlier you detect and treat a developing CTD, the better your chances are of recovering quickly and fully.

By assessing your condition yourself before seeing your doctor, you also will be better prepared to ask questions and to decide whether to accept your doctor's diagnosis or seek a second opinion. For instance, your doctor may not place as much weight as you do on self-reported symptoms and may prefer to rely primarily on electrodiagnostic test results. This chapter will help you to assess your symptoms and, if necessary, to begin preparing for a visit to your doctor.

What Are Your Symptoms?

Before you rush ahead to the more detailed descriptions of CTDs later in this chapter, read the brief description of how your arms and hands work. This will give you important information that will help you understand what happens to you when you develop a CTD.

Your Arms and Hands

Moving from your shoulders down to your fingers, your arms and hands can make increasingly fine movements, but each joint has a smaller range of motion than the preceding one. Your shoulder gives you the freedom to move your arm in any direction, while both your shoulders and your elbows can act as levers, giving strength to arm movements. Your elbow and your wrist together help to rotate your forearm and hand either palm-side up (supination) or palm-side down (pronation). Your wrist bends toward the back of your hand (extension) or toward the palm (flexion), and it is also capable of a modest amount of movement from side to side (radial movement when it bends toward your thumb and ulnar movement when it bends toward your little finger). The joints at the base of your fingers allow you to trace a small circle with your fingertips, while the joints at the tips of your fingers can bend (flex) or straighten (extend).

The shoulder stabilizes and mobilizes the arm, while the arm does the same for the hand and fingers. The bones in your shoulder, arms, and hands bear weight (for example, when you lift something), ligaments in your shoulders and elbows hold the bones together at the joints, and muscles move the bones via tendons that transfer the muscles' force to the bones. The movements your fingers make and the strength in your grip are controlled almost entirely by the muscles in your forearm. The only muscles in your hand are in the base of your thumb. When you want to move your hand, your forearm muscles contract or elongate and your elbow works as a lever to transfer force to the tendons, which in turn move your fingers or hands.

Each tendon is surrounded by synovial fluid encased in a sheath, jointly known as the synovium. Synovial fluid is a lubricant, allowing the tendons to slide through the sheath smoothly and without irritation. In your shoulders and elbows, ligaments and tendon must move over bones. They are protected by sealed, flat sacs filled with synovial fluid called bursae (the singular form is bursa).

Most CTDs occur between the elbows and the fingertips. This region has a high concentration of muscles, tendons, and synovia (plural of synovium) that perform fine and complex movements, making them more vulnerable to irritation and resulting illness than the soft tissues and nerves elsewhere in the body.

When your lower arm, hand, and fingers are doing one motion repeatedly and without an opportunity to rest, or they are placed in an awkward position, the chances increase that you will develop a CTD. The shoulder is vulnerable, particularly in jobs that require you to lift your arms above your head repeatedly, because the muscles in and around it are strong, while the ball-and-socket joint that allows flexibility is unstable, putting considerable stress on the tendons that stabilize it, the rotator cuff tendons.

What are the individual CTDs?

The descriptions of CTDs that follow explain how they develop and what their symptoms are—the information you will need to begin getting a diagnosis of your condition. The discussion of what causes CTDs in Chapter 2 will help you to understand *why* these disorders occur. As you read about CTDs, you may want to make notes about symptoms that you believe apply to you.

This listing of CTDs is organized alphabetically to make it simple for you to find the ailment or ailments you are concerned about. A few of the disorders are much more common than the others, so you might want to start by looking up these five—carpal tunnel syndrome, bursitis, tendinitis, rotator cuff tendinitis, and "tennis elbow" (lateral epicondylitis).*

---

*The medical names for some of these ailments seem less daunting when you know that the suffix "-itis" simply means inflammation.

Screening Techniques You Can Use

To help you and your doctor begin to distinguish among disorders, you can try some simple screening tests. Doing them may help you reach a conclusion about your condition, but doctors do not rely solely on these tests. Think of them as evaluation tools rather than as reliable diagnostic methods.

If you are experiencing pain that you think is due to tentitinits, tenosynovitis, or myositis but are having difficulty determining where, exactly, it is occurring, you can try a series of simple procedures called range of motion maneuvers to help you identify the location. You will need another person to assist you since some of these activities require an "examiner."

One note of warning: If you try these maneuvers, stop immediately if you feel any unusual pain. In some cases, it is possible to harm yourself by continuing.

Passive range of motion maneuvers test for disorders within joints. You should remain passive (making no effort to move) and allow another person to gently bend your joints near the area where the pain seems to be. If you feel pain in the joint, this suggests that the problem may be arthritic or otherwise joint-related. Though passive range of motion maneuvers usually do not indicate CTDs, it is possible to mistake tendon pain *near* a joint for pain *in* the joint.

Resisted range of motion maneuvers can be useful in locating tendinitis, tenosynovitis, myositis, and bursitis. These tests require you to push against resistance provided by your helper. For example, you might raise your arm against your helper's resistance. If the examiner can work out how to offer resistance against motions that involve the muscles and tendons that you suspect are causing your pain, you may be able to isolate the source of your discomfort.

Active range of motion maneuvers allow you to move individual joints freely. For instance, if you can move your shoulder freely and without pain in every direction it will go, both with your fist clenched and with your hand open, you can probably rule out rotator cuff tendinitis.

Bursitis

The bursae that protect the tendons and ligaments in your shoulders and elbows can be irritated and inflamed when you move your shoulder repeatedly and forcefully or when the tissues the bursae protect are themselves swollen or rough. Like all inflamed tissue, bursae can accumulate calcium that subsequently hardens and interferes with movement. If calcified bursitis is allowed to advance, it can restrict motion in the affected joints. Other symptoms include a sensation of grinding, as well as pain that can be sharp.

Bursitis is common, but several physicians note that a high percentage of people who believe they have bursitis actually do not. If you suspect that you have bursitis in the shoulder, you also should ask your doctor about rotator cuff tendinitis or other ailments that are not caused by cumulative trauma.

Screening for Bursitis

You can look for signs of bursitis in three ways: First, try slowly rotating your entire arm at the shoulder joint in a large arc at your side. If you feel pain, this could indicate bursitis. Second, have someone provide gentle resistance as you swing your arm forward, backward, and out to the side from a resting state at your side. This resisted range of motion maneuver requires you to contract the muscles in your shoulder and thus to use the tendons and ligaments there. If the bursae are inflamed, you may feel burning near your shoulder. If the bursitis is calcified, you may also feel a grinding sensation.

Remember that bursitis is commonly confused with rotator cuff tendinitis. Since tendinitis is more likely to feel tender or sore when you press on it, the third screening tool you can use is to push gently with your fingers in the soft areas around your shoulder. If you feel soreness or pain, this makes it less likely that you have bursitis. Of course, it is possible to have both bursitis and rotator cuff tendinitis.

Carpal Tunnel Syndrome

This is the most widely known CTD.

In the wrist (*carpel* in Latin), a set of eight bones

forms a small arch with the opening toward the palm side of your wrist. A strong, stiff ligament, sometimes known as the carpal ligament, covers the opening. The area inside of this structure is the carpal tunnel (see illustration).

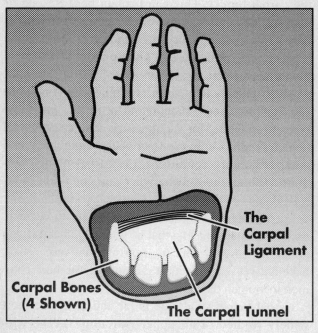

Carpal Bones (4 Shown)

The Carpal Ligament

The Carpal Tunnel

The Carpal Tunnel

Through this tunnel run the tendons and blood vessels going to your hand, as well as the median nerve that provides sensation to the thumb, the pointing finger, the middle finger, and the half of the ring finger next to the middle finger.* The median nerve also supplies sensation to about three-quarters of the palm and the back sides of the three affected fingers.

Carpal tunnel syndrome occurs when the median nerve is compressed or irritated as it passes through the carpal tunnel. This can happen because one or more of the tendons are swollen, because the wrist is bent in a way that reduces the amount of space in the carpal tunnel, or because of a sharp blow to the carpal tunnel area, such as a heavy object falling on your wrist. Swelling and other effects related to conditions such as pregnancy, rheumatoid arthritis, and some types of diabetes, for example, can also cause carpal tunnel syndrome. In cases linked to pregnancy and other temporary conditions, the carpel tunnel syndrome usually goes away when the condition is resolved.

Carpal tunnel syndrome is more likely to occur in your "dominant" hand—that is, your right hand if you are right-handed. And for reasons that researchers have not yet determined, it is significantly more common in women than it is in men.

Carpal tunnel syndrome is far and away the most widely studied of all upper extremity CTDs, with good reason. Though it is less common than tendinitis, carpal tunnel syndrome is arguably the most painful CTD, its symptoms are long-lasting, and it —

---

*It may help you to remember that there are two types of nerves. Sensory nerves provide sensations, such as the ability to feel things in the hand. Motor nerves stimulate and control muscle movements.

Nonoccupational Factors Associated with Carpal Tunnel Syndrome

Age (frequency increases with age)
Arthritis
Diabetes
Gout
Hypothyroidism
Menopause
Pregnancy
Gender (higher frequency in women)
Tumors of tendon sheaths
Use of oral contraceptives
Wrist fractures and dislocations
Wrist size and structure

---

poses a relatively high risk of long-term damage. From a health perspective it is in a different class because it involves a major nerve and so can affect your ability to use your hands. The costs of treating carpal tunnel syndrome, like those of other nerve entrapments, such as ulnar nerve entrapment at the elbow, are consistently higher than other CTDs.

Most doctors and insurance companies accept electrodiagnostic test results as medical confirmation of a carpal tunnel syndrome case, making it easier to study than other CTDs. As a result, much of our knowledge of occupational risk factors associated with CTDs is based on what we have learned about carpal tunnel syndrome. But electrodiagnostic tests detect only those carpal tunnel syndrome cases that have become severe, when treatment is least effective and most expensive. If researchers relied on electrodiagnostic test methods to diagnose carpal tunnel syndrome, we would expect to find only advanced cases in which surgery might be the only option, says NIOSH's Vern Putz-Anderson.

To address this problem, NIOSH has published a case definition to carpal tunnel syndrome (see box) for researchers, which is useful for people evaluating their own conditions. It errs on the side of inclusion to foster an aggressive approach to identifying and treating carpal tunnel syndrome cases before they cause severe, permanent harm.

NIOSH's Definition of a Carpal Tunnel Syndrome Case

A version of the NIOSH definition, modified to simplify medical language, is given below. The definition's either-or construction makes it relatively easy to qualify a case as carpal tunnel syndrome.

A. One or more of the following symptoms suggestive of CTS is present: tingling or burning, decreased feeling, pain, or numbness affecting at least one part of the median nerve distribution of the hand(s). [The median nerve distribution comprises the thumb, the pointing finger, the middle finger, and the side of ring finger nearest to the middle finger, as well as the palm of the thumb side of the hand.] Symptoms should have lasted at least one week or, if intermittent, have occurred on multiple occasions. Other possible causes of numbness and tingling should have been excluded by clinical observation and/or testing.

B. Objective findings consistent with CTS are present in the affected hand(s) and wrist(s). EITHER:
1. Physical examination findings—Either positive results of either Tinel's or Phalen's test (see p. 181) or diminished or absent sensation to pin prick in the median nerve distribution of the hand. OR
2. Electrodiagnostic findings (nerve conduction velocity or electromyography test results) indicative of median nerve dysfunction across the carpal tunnel.

C. Evidence of work-relatedness—a history of a job involving one or more of the following activities preceding the development of symptoms, or pre-existing CTS cases among one or more co-workers performing similar tasks:
1. Frequent, repetitive use of the same or similar movements of the hand or wrist on the affected side(s).
2. Regular tasks requiring the generation of high force by the hand.
3. Regular or sustained tasks requiring awkward hand positions of the affected side(s), such as the pinch grip (used to hold a pencil), extreme flexion, extension, or ulnar deviation of the wrist, and use of the fingers with the wrist flexed.
4. Regular use of vibrating hand-held tools.
5. Frequent or prolonged pressure over the wrist or base of the palm on the affected side(s).

The symptoms commonly associated with carpal tunnel syndrome are:

1. *Tingling, pain, or numbness* in the area of the hand served by the median nerve. Often these sensations first occur while you are sleeping. Many people mistakenly believe this phenomenon occurs because they are sleeping on their hands. Though not everyone with carpal tunnel syndrome has the experience of waking up at night with their hands "on fire," it is probably the best early indicator of a problem even though research has not found a clear explanation for why this symptom is common.

Some people report tingling, pain, or numbness that is not limited to the median nerve area but may feel as if it has spread to the entire lower arm from the elbow down. This could be a result of imprecise observations on their part. It is always a good idea to be as specific as possible in identifying the locations of your own sensations. It also can indicate simultaneous compression of one or both of the other nerves that provide sensation to the arm and hand (see ulnar nerve entrapment at the elbow, ulnar nerve entrapment at the wrist, and thoracic outlet syndrome).

When carpal tunnel syndrome is left untreated, the tingling, pain, or numbness can develop into excruciating pain.

2. *Loss of sensation* can progress rapidly as the median nerve is damaged. Two common effects of this are that you become increasingly clumsy as your ability to feel things in your hands deteriorates and you may have the sensation that your grip has lost strength. This symptom also can occur as decreased sensitivity to hot and cold.

"I have to be careful of hot—anything hot or anything extremely cold—because I can injure myself without knowing it," explains Dorothy Mayes, a former postal worker. This loss of sensitivity comes on gradually, as do all carpal tunnel syndrome symptoms, so it is possible to have a fairly advanced case before you recognize it.

3. *Loss of muscle tone and strength at the base of the thumb* is a sign of advanced carpal tunnel syndrome. This condition is noticeable when the fleshy area at the base of your thumb has atrophied.

Screening for Carpal Tunnel Syndrome

Doctors use two simple tests to screen for carpal tunnel syndrome, and you can do them yourself: *Phalen's maneuver* requires you to put the backs of your hands together with your wrists flexed and your fingers pointing toward the ground (see photo on page 182). Because this forces compression of the median nerve, you will reproduce your symptoms of carpal tunnel syndrome after one minute in this position if you have this disorder. *Tinel's sign* is a simple test in which you rest your hand palm-side up and tap on your wrist where the median nerve passes through. If you experience tingling or numbness in the parts of the hand that receive sensations via the median nerve, you have reason to suspect that you have carpal tunnel syndrome.

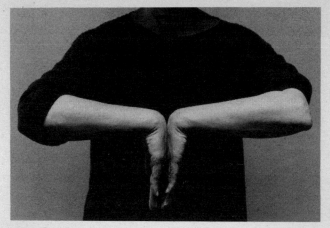

Phalen's Maneuver

Epicondylitis

Epicondylitis is the inflammation or irritation of tendons in the area of an epicondyle, a knucklelike projection at the end of a bone. In the arms, there are two types of epicondylitis—lateral and medial—one for each bump on your elbow.

The tendons in your elbows are unsheathed and are protected against irritation from the bones by bursae. They undergo relatively high levels of physical stress because they are attached to large forearm muscles that control the extension and flexion of your wrists and hands. Movements that involve rotation of the forearm and bending of the wrist at the same time are associated with epicondylitis.

Tennis Elbow *(Lateral epicondylitis)*

Tennis elbow results from rotation of the forearm while extending the wrist, particularly when the movements involve substantial force or repetition—for instance, sanding a piece of wood from side to side. The tendons attached to the muscles that pull your fingers toward the back of your hand get irritated, usually causing pain to extend down the thumb, or lateral, side of your forearm. (This can be confusing, since rotating your forearm can seem to put your thumb on either side of your elbow. For our purposes, assume that your arm is rotated so that the palm of your hand is facing forward with your arm hanging at your side. In this position, your thumb is on the "outside" of your hand, pointing away from your body.)

Lateral epicondylitis is also known as pitcher's elbow and bowler's elbow, indicative of its association with forceful acceleration and deceleration of the arm at the elbow. It is not primarily a sports-related injury, however. It is easy to envision the position of your hand when it is at risk for tennis elbow by pretending you are holding a tennis racket at the peak of its backswing in preparation for a forehand, with your hand fully extended (your wrist pulled back).

Screening for Tennis Elbow

To test for tennis elbow, try to extend your wrist against resistance—a resisted range of motion test. If doing this reproduces your symptoms, it indicates tennis elbow.

Golfer's Elbow (*Medial epicondylitis*)

Golfer's elbow differs from tennis elbow in that it involves the tendons that connect the knob on the inside (medial side) of your elbow to the muscles that flex the hand. To experience the type of movement that would put your arm at risk for golfer's elbow, try using an imaginary scoop to pick up a scoopful of sand. Reach your arm directly in front of you and then pull the scoop down and toward you, curling it up when it gets near your body.

Screening for Golfer's Elbow

The test for golfer's elbow is similar to the one for tennis elbow. Flex your wrist against resistance. If this produces your symptoms, you probably have golfer's elbow.

Myositis

Excessive or improper use of a muscle can cause it to become inflamed, a condition called myositis. Myositis is considered a CTD only when it results from repetitive use over time. Any muscle can be affected, though large muscles such as the biceps are more probable sites than are small muscles. A pulled or strained muscle resulting from an isolated incident, such as wrenching your wrist, would not be classified as a CTD.

Screening for Myositis

Most people are familiar with the feeling of a sore muscle. It aches. If the muscle is injured (for example, torn), the pain is noticeably sharper. A resisted range of movement maneuver that involved a muscle you feel may be inflamed will produce or increase the aching sensation if you have myositis. If the illness has occurred in a muscle near a tendon, it may be difficult to isolate the disorder.

Raynaud's Syndrome

As an occupational illness, Raynaud's syndrome (occasionally called Raynaud's disease) is most often associated with prolonged use of vibrating equipment such as a jackhammer or a pneumatic tool. In Raynaud's syndrome, the flow of blood to your hands is reduced by constricting blood vessels. The cause of the constriction may be overstimulation of the nerves in the hand and arm, but researchers cannot agree on whether this or other factors explain the phenomenon. It is not unusual for Raynaud's syndrome to develop in people with advanced cases of carpal tunnel syndrome, and it is also common among people with connective tissue diseases such as some types of lupus. (Though the term *Raynaud's phenomenon* is no longer commonly used, you may still hear it on occasion when Raynaud's syndrome accompanies a connective tissue disease.) People with Raynaud's syndrome often develop pale, white, or blue hands, particularly following exposure to the cold. Their hands often are unusually sensitive to cold. Occasionally, Raynaud's syndrome produces tingling or numbness in the hands, and in extreme cases can lead to the loss of sensation in or control of the fingers.

Screening for Raynaud's Syndrome

There are no tests for Raynaud's syndrome. While the symptoms are usually clear, physicians rely solely on the patient's symptoms and health history.

Tendinitis

Tendinitis (sometimes tendonitis) is the most common type of CTD. Every time you contract a muscle, you put strain on the tendon that connects that muscle to a bone. Repeated contractions over an extended period can cause the tendon to fray or tear. This makes the tendon rough and inflamed, increasing the friction that is wearing away at it. In your shoulder and elbow, where the tendons are unsheathed, calcium deposits sometimes form. These can further irritate the condition, cause increasingly sharp pain, and produce a grinding feeling in the affected joint. Calcified tendinitis usually will restrict the tendon's ability to move freely. When the tendon is in use, the pain from tendinitis can be sharp. Often when the tendon is not in use, it aches. Unless the tendon is allowed to heal before it is severely damaged, it may be irreparably weakened.

Screening for Tendinitis

The best methods of testing for tendinitis are the range of motion maneuvers described earlier. Passive range of motion maneuvers should produce no pain, active range of motion maneuvers may if the movement involves the affected tendon, and resisted range of motion maneuvers are most likely to cause pain *if the resistance is applied in a way that effectively isolates the affected tendon.*

Rotator Cuff Tendinitis

The tendons from four sets of muscles join together in your shoulder to give the joint stability and mobility. Because they are unsheathed and because they are strained most severely by jerky movements or forceful activities that require that the elbow be raised, it is easy to understand why baseball pitchers often are beset by rotator cuff injuries. Swimmers also are at risk for rotator cuff tendinitis. Still, nonathletes can and do develop rotator cuff tendinitis routinely. This disorder is more common in people over sixty years of age. A rotator cuff *tear,* a more severe disorder, occurs when one, or more, of the four tendons is torn to a significant degree. While the major tear usually results from a single motion, such as pitching a baseball, the tendon probably is already torn or frayed from repeated stress.

Like all tendinitis, rotator cuff tendinitis more often causes constant aching than stabbing pains. But the pain can be sharp, particularly at night. People with rotator cuff tendinitis often suspect that they have bursitis.

Screening for Rotator Cuff Tendinitis

To screen for possible rotator cuff tendinitis, first see whether you can rotate your entire arm in a wide circle without pain or weakness. This is a simple, active range of motion maneuver. You can also try a test that doctors use: With the thumb on the side of the affected shoulder, trace a line up your lower spine. You should not feel any unusual pain, in your shoulder even when pressing the thumb up your spine with your other hand. If you do experience pain, stop immediately.

Tenosynovitis

Tenosynovitis occurs when the sheathing, or synovium, through which your tendons glide is injured or overused, producing an excess of synovial fluid, a lubricant. If this fluid collects, the synovium swells and loses some of its ability to function. This can produce pain in the affected area.

Screening for Tenosynovitis

Use range of motion maneuvers to look for symptoms. Start by identifying the area where you think the tenosynovitis may have developed, and see if you can figure out a motion that causes the sensation you have been feeling. In effect, you are doing an active range of motion maneuver. Next, try the same movement using a resisted range of motion maneuver. This should also produce the sensation. A passive range of motion maneuver in which the person working with you moves your hand or arm for you using the same motion can rule out the possibility of a joint disorder, as long as this maneuver produces no pain.

Ganglion Cyst

When the snyovium surrounding a tendon is repeatedly and persistently rubbed or pressed in one spot, it can swell with synovial fluid and produce a ball-like bump that shows through your skin. This type of tenosynovitis is most often seen at the base of the hand where tendons pass near the carpal bones. Test for this by resting your hand on the bone while moving your fingers, particularly your little finger. In this way you put pressure on the tendon, increasing the chances of irritating the synovium. Ganglion, or knot-like, cysts are easy to identify visually and rarely produce significant pain.

Stenosing Tenosynovitis

Sometimes the swelling synovium progressively compresses the tendon it is supposed to protect and lubricate. This is known as a stenosing tenosynovitis (stenosis is the narrowing or tightening of a passageway).

De Quervain's Disease

When stenosing tenosynovitis involves the tendons at the base and the side of the thumb, it is called De Quervain's disease (or De Quervain's syndrome or disorder). The two tendons that control the thumb's movement share a synovium, and this is where the problem occurs. In addition to aching around the base of the thumb, it can produce thumb weakness and decreased tone in the muscles on the top of the forearm that extend the wrist.

Screening for De Quervain's Disease

The standard screening test doctors use for De Quervain's disease is called Finkelstein's test. To do this yourself, fold your thumb across the palm of your hand and wrap your fingers firmly over your thumb (see photo). Bend your wrist in the direction of your little finger. If this position produces pain or aching in

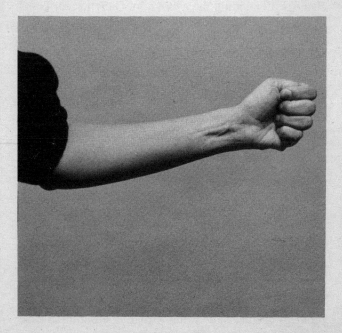

Finkelstein's Test

the base of your thumb, that is considered a sign that you have De Quervain's disease.

Trigger finger *(Stenosing tenosynovitis crepitans)*

In severe cases, the stenosis reaches an extreme condition and the tendon is locked in place, unable to move except in uneven, jerky leaps. This is commonly known as trigger finger. In addition to pain in the forearm and either finger stiffness or jerky finger movements, stenosing tenosynovitis crepitans can produce a crackling sound as the tendon grinds through the synovium.

Thoracic Outlet Syndrome

The nerves and blood vessels exiting the torso to the arms must pass through a confined space between your collarbone and your uppermost rib. This space is called the thoracic outlet. Any sustained position or repetitive movement such as holding your arms above your head that reduces the size of the space can compress either the nerves or the blood vessels, or both.

Both the median and ulnar nerves can be affected, causing tingling or numbness in the fingers and hands, weakened hands, arm pain, and deterioration of muscles in the hands and forearms. It is sometimes possible to learn which of the nerves is affected by determining which part of the hand and forearm are symptomatic. The ulnar nerve supplies the little finger and half of the ring finger, as well as the side of the forearm nearest the little finger. The median nerve supplies the rest of the fingers.

Pressure on the blood vessels passing through the thoracic outlet reduces the blood flow to and from the tendons, ligaments, and muscles. This reduces the amount of oxygen and nutrients these tissues receive, as well as the amount of tissue waste the blood removes, decreasing the ability of muscles, in particular, to recover from exertion and to work for extended periods. Reduced blood flow can produce pale, white, and blue hands (as with Raynaud's syndrome), and chronically tired arms.

In the medical community, thoracic outlet syndrome is one of the more controversial CTDs. There is considerable disagreement about whether the symptoms are caused by compression of the nerves or compression of the blood vessels, since the two pass through the thoracic outlet together.

Screening for Thoracic Outlet Syndrome

Doctors will use a series of maneuvers to compare your nerve responses and blood flow when your arm is in different positions. You can try one of them.

With your arm resting in your lap, take your pulse. Then raise your arm straight above your head with your hand reaching for the sky and take your pulse again (or have another person take your pulse in this position). Thoracic outlet syndrome can make your pulse much weaker in the second position. If it is extreme, you may not be able to feel your pulse at all.

Thoracic outlet syndrome is particularly difficult to diagnose because it can involve the nerves, the blood vessels, or both. The screening test described here is less reliable than those explained for other CTDs in this chapter. If this test does not produce a weaker pulse, this does not mean you can rule out thoracic outlet syndrome. You still may want to visit your doctor.

Ulnar Nerve Entrapment at the Elbow

When the ulnar nerve is compressed for an extended period at the elbow, the resulting sensation can be similar to what you feel when you bump your "funny bone"—tingling and numbness in your little finger and part of your ring finger. Some cases also produce significant pain in this area. The sensations often are strongest during the night. This condition used to be called "telephone operator's arm" and is sometimes still called "beer drinker's arm," in recognition of the tendency of people to rest their elbows on bars. Over time, unresolved unlar entrapment at the elbow can weaken your grip.

Screening for Ulnar Nerve Entrapment at the Elbow

You can test for ulnar nerve entrapment at the elbow (sometimes called cubital outlet syndrome) by tapping on the ulnar nerve where it passes through your elbow (the cubital tunnel), much as you would test for Tinel's sign at the wrist for carpal tunnel syndrome.

With your elbow bent and your forearm lightly supported, have someone tap on the "funny bone" soft spot of your elbow. If this produces symptomatic sensations in your little finger and ring finger, you may have ulnar entrapment at the elbow.

Ulnar Nerve Entrapment at the Wrist

The ulnar nerve, which supplies the little finger and half of the ring finger, as well the back of the hand, passes through the wrist to the little-finger side of the carpal tunnel at a location called Guyon's tunnel. Like the median nerve, it can be compressed or entrapped by swelling, but more commonly it is affected by prolonged or repeated ulnar deviation—bending the wrist in the direction of the little finger. The primary symptom of this ulnar nerve entrapment (also known as Guyon's tunnel syndrome and Guyon's canal syndrome) is weakness in the hand. Unlike the sensations that accompany carpal tunnel syndrome, ulnar nerve entrapment at the wrist does not produce tingling, numbness, or pain because the branch of the ulnar nerve that supplies feelings branches off above the wrist and does not pass through Guyon's tunnel. Ulnar nerve entrapment at the elbow or at the shoulder (as part of thoracic outlet syndrome) *can* cause both these sensations and weakness in the hand.

Screening for Ulnar Nerve Entrapment at the Wrist

Because this condition is marked by loss of muscle strength, the simplest screening test is a resisted motion maneuver in which the person helping you offers resistance while you try to curl your little finger and ring finger into your palm. For comparison, do this with both hands.

GLOSSARY

Bursa—Sealed, flat sacs filled with fluid that protect ligaments and tendons in your shoulders and elbows where they must move over bones.

Brachial plexus—A cablelike structure that comprises the major nerves and blood vessels into your arm. The brachial plexus passes through the thoracic outlet.

BLS (Bureau of Labor Statistics)—The office within the Department of Labor that gathers, analyzes, and publishes data on, among other topics, the number of occupational illnesses and injuries that occur each year.

Carpal tunnel—A structure in your wrist made up of eight bones that form a small arch with the opening toward the palm side of your wrist. A strong, stiff ligament, sometimes known as the carpal ligament, covers the opening.

Cubital outlet—The passageway in the elbow that the ulnar nerve passes through.

Electromyography (EMG)—A method of measuring the responses of muscles to electrical stimuli.

Epicondyle—A knucklelike projection at the end of a bone.

Ergonomics—The science of fitting machines and equipment to the people who use them.

Ganglion—A ball-like bump or cyst produced by pooling of synovial fluid.

Guyon's canal—The passageway in the wrist that the ulnar nerve passes through.

Ligament—A kind of soft tissue that connects bones to bones.

Median nerve—The nerve that provides sensation to the thumb, the pointing finger, the middle finger, and the half of the ring finger next to the middle finger, as well as about three-quarters of the palm and the back sides of the three affected fingers.

Nerve conduction velocity—The speed at which a nerve signal travels. A damaged nerve transmits the signal at a slower than normal speed.

NIOSH—The National Institute for Occupational

Safety and Health, the federal agency primarily responsible for research on work-related safety and health. NIOSH is part of the Centers for Disease Control, which is in turn part of the Department of Health and Human Services.

OSHA—The Occupational Safety and Health Administration, the federal agency primarily responsible for regulation of work-related safety and for enforcing regulations. OSHA is part of the Department of Labor.

Pronation—Rotating your hand and forearm palm down.

Radial deviation—Bending your wrist in the direction of your thumb.

Rotator cuff—Four sets of muscles working together in your shoulder to give the joint stability and mobility.

Shoulder abduction—Moving your arm from the shoulder out to your side, such as when you point to the side with your hand with your arm at a right angle to your body.

Shoulder adduction—Pulling in your arm at the shoulder, such as when you hunch your shoulder.

Shoulder extension—Moving your arm from the shoulder so that it is behind you.

Shoulder flexion—Moving your arm from the shoulder so that it is in front of you.

Stenosis—The narrowing or tightening of a passageway.

Supination—Rotating your hand and forearm palm up.

Synovitis—Inflammation of the sheath and fluid surrounding the tendon.

Tendon—A kind of soft tissue that connects your muscles to your bones.

Thoracic outlet—A confined space between your collarbone and your uppermost rib.

Ulnar deviation—Bending your wrist in the direction of your little finger.

Ulnar nerve—The nerve that supplies sensation to your little finger and half of your ring finger, as well as the side of your forearm nearest your little finger.

Vibrometry—A relatively new method of testing for nerve damage in which multiple vibration frequencies are applied to one of your fingers. The finger selected is one of those that gets its sensation from the nerve that appears to be damaged.

Wrist extension—Bending your wrist in the direction of the back of your hand.

Wrist flexion—Bending your wrist in the direction of your palm.

REFERENCES

Anderson, H., M. Cullen, E. Eisen, R. Feldman, J. Hughes, M. J. Jacobs, K. Kriess, J. Melius, J. Peters, and D. Wegman. "From the Centers for Disease Control: Occupational Disease Surveillance: Carpal Tunnel Syndrome," *Journal of the American Medical Association, 262*(7), 886, 889. August 18, 1989.

Armstrong, Thomas J., Ph.D. "an Ergonomics Guide to Carpal Tunnel Syndrome." *American Industrial Hygiene Association Journal*, 1983.

Armstrong, Thomas J., and Yair Lifshitz. "Evaluation and Design of Jobs for Control of Cumulative Trauma Disorders." In *Ergonomic Interventions to Prevent Musculoskeletal Injuries in Industry,* (pp. 73–85). Chelsea, MI: Lewis Publishers, 1987.

Bertolini, Renzo. *Carpal Tunnel Syndrome: A Summary of the Occupational Health Concern* (Report No. P90-6E; 2nd ed.). Canadian Centre for Occupational Safety and Health, 1992.

"Comprehensive Occupational Safety and Health Reform Act." Hearings before the Subcommittee on Labor and the Committee on Labor and Human Resources, U.S. Senate, March 17, May 6, and June 10, 1992.

"Confronting Repetitive Motion Illnesses in the Workplace." Hearing before the Employment and Housing Subcommittee of the Committee on Government Operations, U.S. House of Representatives, March 28, 1991.

Cotton, Paul. "Symptoms May Return After Carpal Tunnel Surgery." *Journal of the American Medical Association,* 265(15), 1922–25, April 17, 1991.

Dainoff, Marvin J., and Marilyn Hecht Dainoff. *People & Productivity.* Toronto, Ontario: Holt, Rinehart and Winston, 1986.

Dickerson, O. Bruce. "Medical Aspects of Cumulative Trauma Disorders." In *Cumulative Trauma Disorders in the Workplace: Costs, Prevention, and Progress,* (pp. 123–136). Washington, DC: Bureau of National Affairs.

Eccleston, Stacey M., ed. *The Americans with Disabilities Act: Implications for Workers' Compensation.*

Cambridge, MA: Workers Compensation Research Institute, 1992.

Fihn, Stephan, and Steven McGee. *Outpatient Medicine*. Philadelphia: W. B. Saunders, 1992.

Glane, Walter D., Kenneth N. Anderson, and Lois E. Anderson. *The Signet/Mosby Medical Encyclopedia*. New York: Signet, 1987.

Hadler, Nortin M., "Arm Pain in the Workplace: A Small Area Analysis," *Journal of Occupational Medicine, 34*(2), February 1992.

The Human Factors Society (ANSI/HFS 100-1988). Santa Monica, CA, 1988.

Jetzer, Thomas C. "Use of Vibration Testing in the Early Evaluation of Workers with Carpal Tunnel Syndrome." *Journal of Occupational Medicine, 33(2)*, 117–120, February, 1991.

Kapit, Wynn, and Lawrence M. Elson. *The Anatomy Coloring Book*. New York: Harper & Row, 1977.

Karasek, Robert. "Job Decision Latitude, Job Design, and Coronary Heart Disease." In G. Salvendy and M. J. Smith, eds., *Machine Pacing and Occupational Stress*. London: Taylor & Francis, 1981.

Karasek, Robert, and Tores Theorell. *Health Work: Stress, Productivity, and the Reconstruction of Working Life*. New York: Basic Books, 1990.

Katz, Jeffrey N., Martin G. Larson, Amin Subra,

Christian Krarup, Craig R. Stirrat, Rajesh Sethi, Holley M. Eaton, Anne H. Fossel, and Matthew H. Liang. "The Carpal Tunnel Syndrome: Diagnostic Utility of the History and Physical Examination Findings." *Annals of Internal Medicine, 112,* 321–327.

Marras, William S. *An Ergonomic Analysis of the LSM and FSM Operations in the U.S. Post Office.* Washington, DC: Occupational Safety and Health Administration, 1991.

Murley, A. G. H., 1975, "The Painful Elbow," *Practitioner, 215,* 36–41.

Nancollas, Michael P., Clayton A. Peimar, and Dale R. Wheeler. "Long-term Results of Carpal Tunnel Release." Presented to the 1991 meeting of the American Academy of Orthopaedic Surgeons, Anaheim, CA. Also reported in Cotton, 1991.

Nathan, P. A., K. D. Meadows, and Linda S. Doyle. "Occupation as a Risk Factor for Impaired Sensory Conduction of the Median Nerve at the Carpal Tunnel." *The Journal of Hand Surgery, 13-B*(2), 167–170, May 1988.

Occupational Safety and Health Administration, "Ergonomic Safety and Health Management" (Advanced Notice of Proposed Rulemaking). *Federal Register, 57,* No. 149, August 3, 1992, pp. 34192–34200.

Pagnanelli, David M. and Steven J. Barrer. "Carpal Tunnel Syndrome: Surgical Treatment Using the

Paine Retinaculatome." *Journal of Neurosurgery, 75,* 77–81, July 1991.

Putz-Anderson, Vern, ed. *Cumulative Trauma Disorders: A Manual for Musculoskeletal Diseases of the Upper Limbs,* Bristol, PA: Taylor & Francis, 1988.

Putz-Anderson, Vern. "The Impact of Automation on Musculoskeletal Disorders." In *Ergonomics of Hybrid Automated Systems I,* Karwowski et al., ed. Amsterdam: Elsevier Science Publishers, 1988.

Rempel, David M., Robert J. Harrison, and Scott Barnhart. "Work-Related Cumulative Trauma Disorders of the Upper Extremity (Special Communication)." *Journal of the American Medical Association, 267*(6), 838–842, February 12, 1992.

Schottland, John R., Gordon J. Kirschberg, Roger Fillingim, Voris P. Davis, and Fran Hogg. "Median Nerve Latencies in Poultry Processing Workers: An Approach to Resolving the Role of Industrial 'Cumulative Trauma' in the Development of Carpal Tunnel Syndrome." *Journal of Occupational Medicine, 33*(5), 627–631, 1991.

Silverstein, Barbara A, Lawrence J. Fine, and Thomas J. Armstrong. "Occupational Factors and Carpal Tunnel Syndrome." *American Journal of Industrial Medicine* (Vol. 11, pp. 343–358), 1987.

Silverstein, Michael. Letter to the editor. *Journal of Occupational Medicine, 34*(11), 119–120, November 1992.

Taylor, W. *The Vibration Syndrome*. New York: Academic Press, 1974.

Winn, Francis J., and Vern Putz-Anderson. "Vibration Thresholds as a Function of Age and Diagnosis of Carpal Tunnel Syndrome: A Preliminary Report." *Experimental Aging Research, 16*(4), 221–224, November 4, 1990.

The information presented in this book is intended to help you better understand and cope with cumulative trauma disorders of the upper extremities. This book has been reviewed by qualified physicians. It can be a valuable addition to your doctor's advice, and it should be used under his or her care and direction. The author and publisher disclaim all responsibility for any adverse effects resulting from the information contained herein.

This book is not intended as a substitute for medical advice. The reader should regularly consult a physician or health care professional in matters relating to health and particularly in respect to any symptoms that may require diagnosis or medical attention.

Photographs by Stephen Perloff